Dosage Forms - Innovation and Future Perspectives

Edited by Usama Ahmad

Published in London, United Kingdom

Dosage Forms - Innovation and Future Perspectives
http://dx.doi.org/10.5772/intechopen.95734
Edited by Usama Ahmad

Contributors
Marouene Bejaoui, Salah Kouass, Haykel Galai, Fathi Touati, Alaa Yehya, Rajesh Sonti, Siva Nageswara Rao Gajula, Amol G Dikundwar, Sakina Vora, Sunil T. Galatage, Rahul Trivedi, Durgacharan A. Bhagwat, Arehalli S. Manjappa, Swapnil S. Harale, Abhinandan A. Alman, Swapnil S. Chopade, Sujit A. Desai, Shashikant Adsul, Ashish M. Phutane, Samruddhi S. Kadam, Shruti R. Mandekar, Amruta M. Chougale, Krushnabai R. Margale, Rohini M. Patil, Shweta N. Kalebere, Amolkumar A. Kempwade, Muthukumar Subramanian, Gayathri Rajaram, Vinesha Ravi, Chellam Sankar, Fikadu Ejeta, Shubham Thakur, Palvi Sharma, Ritika Sharma, Ankita Rajput, Inampudi Sailaja, Pooja Pawar, Ivvala Anand Shaker, Tomislav Katanec, Dragana Gabrić

First published in London, United Kingdom, 2023 by IntechOpen
IntechOpen is the global imprint of INTECHOPEN LIMITED, registered in England and Wales, registration number: 11086078, 5 Princes Gate Court, London, SW7 2QJ, United Kingdom

British Library Cataloguing-in-Publication Data
A catalogue record for this book is available from the British Library

Additional hard and PDF copies can be obtained from orders@intechopen.com

Dosage Forms - Innovation and Future Perspectives
Edited by Usama Ahmad
p. cm.
Print ISBN 978-1-80355-210-1
Online ISBN 978-1-80355-211-8
eBook (PDF) ISBN 978-1-80355-212-5

Meet the editor

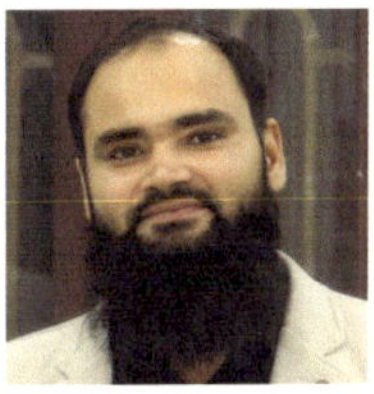

Dr. Usama Ahmad holds a specialization in Pharmaceutics from Amity University, Lucknow, India. He received his Ph.D. in 2018 from Integral University, Lucknow, India. Currently, he is an Associate Professor of Pharmaceutics, at the Faculty of Pharmacy, Integral University. From 2013 to 2014 he worked on a research project funded by the Science and Engineering Research Board, Department of Science and Technology (SERB-DST), Government of India. He has a rich publication record with more than twenty-seven original journal articles, five edited books, nine book chapters, and several scientific articles to his credit. He is a member of the American Association for Cancer Research, the International Association for the Study of Lung Cancer, and the British Society for Nanomedicine. Dr. Ahmad's research focus is on the development of nanoformulations to facilitate the delivery of drugs.

Contents

Preface

Dosage forms, also known as drug delivery systems, are an essential aspect of modern pharmaceutical science. They are the physical forms in which drugs are administered to patients and they play a crucial role in determining the efficacy and safety of a medication. The field of dosage forms is vast and diverse, encompassing everything from traditional solid and liquid forms to newer technologies such as nanoparticles and gene therapy.

This book provides detailed explanations of the various technologies and techniques used to develop dosage forms and examines some of the dosage forms used in modern pharmaceutical science. It also examines progress and highlights recent developments in the field. Furthermore, the book highlights the practical aspects of dosage forms, including their formulation and development.

Chapter 1, 'Layered Tablets: A Novel Oral Solid Dosage Form', highlights the importance of layered tablets and how patient compliance can be improved by reducing the number of tablets administered to patients at one time. Chapter 2, 'Orally Disintegrating Tablets', discusses the production of tablets that have rapid disintegration in the oral cavity. Chapter 3, 'Multifunctional Roles of PVP as a Versatile Biomaterial in Solid State', examines the multifunctional role of Polyvinylpyrrolidone (PVP) in the solid state and demonstrates how PVP made it possible to overcome several challenges in drug formulations, such as solubility and bioavailability weakness, physical instability under stress conditions, and complexation efficiency of cyclodextrin molecules. Chapter 4, 'Self-nano Emulsifying Formulations: An Encouraging Approach for Bioavailability Enhancement and Future Perspective', provides valuable information on lipid-based lipid-based formulations for increasing the bioavailability of poorly soluble drugs. Chapter 5, 'Novel Topical Drug Delivery Systems in Ophthalmic Applications', examines the progress made in novel dosage forms meant for delivery to the eyes. Chapter 6, 'Interplay between Pharmacokinetics and Pharmacogenomics', provides in-depth information on how an individual's genetic makeup can be the key to creating personalized drugs with greater efficacy and safety. It describes how polymorphism may alter the pharmacokinetic properties of administered drugs. Chapter 7, '*In Vitro* Drug Metabolism Studies Using Human Liver Microsomes', explains why understanding the metabolic stability and kinetics of glucuronidation of an investigational drug is crucial for predicting the pharmacokinetic parameters that support dosing and dose frequency. It provides detailed information about metabolite profiling, metabolic stability, glucuronidation kinetics, reactive metabolites identification, CYP enzyme inhibition, and general protocols using human liver microsomes. Chapter 8, 'Use of Statins in Dental Implantology and Their Impact on Osseointegration: Animal Studies', discusses the relationship between local use of statins and better osseointegration. Finally, Chapter 9, 'Perspective Chapter: Tuberculosis Drugs Doses from Indian Scenario – A Review', presents research on tuberculosis treatment in India in recent years with the goal of providing advice to healthcare providers.

The goal of this book is to provide readers with a solid understanding of the scientific and technological principles that underlie the development of dosage forms. By providing a thorough introduction to the field and its key concepts, the book aims to equip readers with the knowledge and skills needed to understand the latest research and developments in the field as well as to pursue careers in pharmaceutical science or related fields.

Overall, this book is an essential resource for anyone interested in the field of dosage forms, including students, researchers, and practitioners in pharmaceutical science, pharmacy, and medicine. With its detailed explanations and practical examples it provides a comprehensive and accessible introduction to this complex and rapidly evolving field.

Usama Ahmad
Faculty of Pharmacy,
Department of Pharmaceutics,
Integral University,
Lucknow, India

Section 1

Solid Dosage Forms and Role of Excipients

Chapter 1

Layered Tablets: A Novel Oral Solid Dosage Form

Muthukumar Subramanian, Chellam Sankar, Gayathri Rajaram and Vinesha Ravi

Abstract

Oral solid dosage forms hold a predominant position in the drug delivery system. Tablets are the most widely used and convenient dosage form. Due to their ease of manufacturing, the minimum cost of production, easy handling and storage, and better stability, tablets are most preferred. Patients who are prescribed more than one drug are in a situation to consume multiple tablets. To minimize the counts, one or more drugs are cast into layers to form a single tablet, thus called layered tablets. Layered tablets tend to improve patient compliance and reduce the cost of production by half. Layers can be of multiple drugs or the same drug at different doses or drugs with release enhancers or drugs with fillers. Layered tablets hold a greater potential with better patient outcomes as well as stay production-friendly.

Keywords: Oral solid dosage form, layered tablets, compliance, release enhancers

1. Introduction

A particular route of administration is conferred to a drug therapy based on its intended site of action, physicochemical properties, targeting aspects, the convenience of administration, stability, duration and onset of action, and many others. All these parameters help in building a stable, efficient, and therapeutically sound product. The most commonly used routes of administration include oral, IV, IM, and transdermal.

Since the era of drug delivery, the oral dosage is retaining an unbeatable position in drug administration. A drug delivery system aims at improving the efficiency of the treatment and various parameters like handling, administration, storage, etc. The oral route of drug administration is one of the oldest choices and has been consistently dominating the world of drug delivery. It comes with enormous merits like improved patient compliance, a simple manufacturing process, less complex requirements, easy storage and handling, and so on. Despite hindrances like first-pass metabolism, slow onset of action compared to IV/IM, and recent advances in novel drug delivery, the oral solid dosage form has still not lost its dominance.

The oral route is the most widely accepted and marketed route of administration. Besides convenience, it gives the advantage of enhanced absorption. The gastrointestinal tract has a larger surface area conferring to increased absorption of drugs. The intestinal epithelial wall is composed of villi, a micro- erective structure, that increases the absorptive surface area in the gastrointestinal tract up to 300–400 m^2 [1]. Pharmaceutical active ingredients are mostly weak acids or weak bases. The absorption of drugs is based on pH and dissociation constant. Drugs exhibit various degrees of absorption at differing pH. GIT offers a wide range of pH from highly acidic to highly basic nature (0.8–8). This enables absorption of both acidic and basic drugs. The stomach is a primary organ for the absorption of acidic drugs. The intestine has a grading basic pH enhancing the absorption of basic drugs [2, 3].

The oral dosage form denotes systems administered by the oral route. Being the most anticipated route, many formulations are available in the market. They can be solids, liquids, and semi-solids. One of the major factors to be considered for developing a formulation is its pharmaceutical stability. Solids showcase high mechanical, microbial, and chemical stability. An added advantage of oral solids is they do not require sterile manufacturing needs. No much sophistication is needed for manufacturing. Simple instruments are sufficient to produce large quantities of oral solids.

Commonly seen oral solids are tablets, capsules, and pellets. Oral solids are non-invasive and stand out due to its higher compliance and accepted for long term therapy. Production cost of oral solids are lower with retail price remains affordable too. Mechanical strength makes it easier to handle, transport and store. They can also provide modified release of drug enabling sustained, controlled and immediate release.

Despite all these advantages, oral solids bear some disadvantages. Solids are not a preferred dosage form for geriatric and pediatric patients. Dysphagic patients find it difficult to swallow solids and it is not an option for unconscious patient. Even with immediate release mechanism, it takes a lag time to disintegrate, dissolve and reach systemic circulation. It may take some to initiate onset of action, making it not an option for emergency conditions. One unavoidable hinderance is first pass metabolism. GIT is a high degradative pathway conferring to presence to enzymes, acid secretions and altering transit time. Recent advancements like oro-dispersible tablets and sublingual tablets are available, but still oral solids are not comparable to parenteral.

2. Tablets

Tablets are popularly denoted as unit dosage form is an which contains active ingredient(s) and excipients, compressed into a compact solid. It is available in various shapes like, circular, cylindrical, triangular. They are mostly circular, with convex ends and blunt edges. Tablets are manufactured by compressing the actives and other ingredients by use of punches and dies. Tablets may carry break line, break marks and symbols for breaking and identification. They are usually swallowed with liquids, may be chewable, oral disintegrating, etc.....

Tablets are unit dosage form that offers accurate dosing at an affordable price. With increased consumption, simple large-scale production makes it more feasible. Other advantages include easy and cost-effective handling, and ease of identification, as tablets come in various shapes, sizes and colors.

Tableting may be affected by due to the poor compressibility and flow properties of powders which is a major compression parameter. The minimum dose also plays a role in compression. Unacceptable taste and odour make it difficult to devise formulation. Physical instability is a serious drawback that can affect the formulation which could be overcome by encapsulation.

In order to classify the tablets representatively, a schematic flow chart is shown in **Figure 1**.

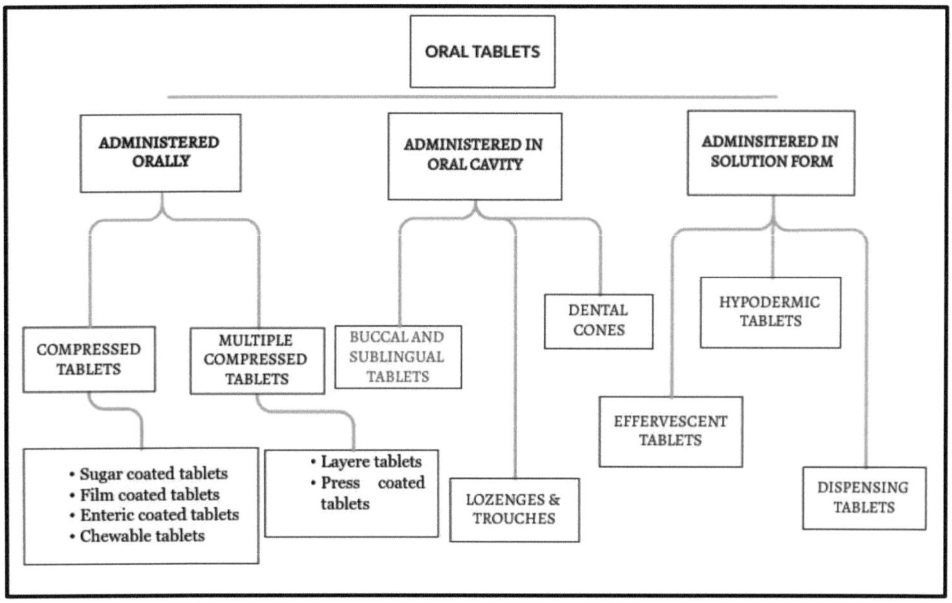

Figure 1.
Flow chart of types of tablets.

3. Layered tablets

The layered tablet is a combination of one or more APIs (Active Pharmaceutical Ingredients) along with excipients, cast in two or more layers to form a single unit dosage form. Formulating a combination of drugs in a single dosage form is appreciated in the case of long-term therapy like parkinsonism [4]. The noticeable feature is that the drug is released without any pharmacokinetic interactions with individual release rate [5]. It can greatly help in minimizing the dosing frequency and can also add to the synergistic effect [6].

The ideal properties expected for a layered tablet include sufficient mechanical strength, better chemical, and physical stability, and no interaction between the layers. The layered tablets exhibit increased patient compliance as the dosing burden is reduced [7]. Layers of the tablet can provide multiple release kinetics of the same or different drugs of the same or different physicochemical properties and showcase different release control mechanisms [8]. Generally, when two or more drugs are co-administered, they might possess the ability to enhance the effect of each other. The layered tablets are the potential in offering such a synergistic effect [6, 9]. These layered tablets also confer high product identification, as the layers are usually of different colours and enable patients to identify the tablets at ease. This also contributes to the attractive appearance of the dosage form.

The bigger advantage is that dual release profiles are obtained in a single unit dosage form. One layer can promote immediate release while the other may contribute to controlled or sustained release [10]. It is very much possible to avoid active-active, active – excipient and excipient - excipient interactions. The cost of production is reduced to a greater extent as the production of two or more tablets is merged into one. It is time-saving and production-friendly.

Accurate dosing and minimized inter-unit variability make it a potential candidate. Low production cost helps in reducing health care expenditure. Ease of packing and handling are added advantages. For a patient under multiple drug regimens, it is easier to carry a single unit compared to multiple units. For drugs with bitter/ obnoxious taste, the oral route may be less preferred. This can be overcome by adapting various taste-masking techniques. Incompatibility is a serious issue when various drugs are administered together. Two incompatible drugs can be administered together by adding an inert layer between the active layers [8]. Fillers constitute a majority of a tablet. When two or more drugs are administered in a single dosage form, there is a possible reduction in the use of excipients like fillers. Layered tablets are very much preferred in case of multiple drug therapy and long-term care.

When it comes to the disadvantages, the weight of the tablet remains a major concern. With all the fillers and inert separating layers, weight adjustment of each layer during a continuous batch is difficult. The layers should have sufficient binding capacity to hold the formulation together. This requires high throughput planning and pre-formulation. Lack of binding of two or more layers and separation of layers. High labor input and equipment sophistication are necessary. Based on the active ingredients, layered tablets are classified as bi-layered tablets with a single active ingredient or bi-layered with two different active ingredients. Tri-layered tablets have three different active ingredients. Based on formulation type, bi-layered tablets may contain one immediate release and another sustained-release layer; two immediate layers; one sustained release and another inert supporting layer; one sustained-release and another inert protecting layer.

4. Release aspect

These bi-layered to multi-layered tablets are formulated to achieve desired release kinetics such as immediate-release, controlled release based on time, pH and related factors, zero-order sustained release, etc. [11, 12]. Bi-layered tablets comprise an immediate-release layer and another extended-release layer. The immediate-release layer disintegrates immediately on reaching the GIT and releases a loading dose. While the other layer stays for a longer period in GIT and maintains drug plasma concentration. The hydrophobic/hydrophilic polymer matrix layer in layered tablets is used in controlling the drug release pattern by hydrophobic polymer coating over the hydrophilic matrix to attain sustained release, whereas one-sided coating aid in controlled release of the drug. In the case of a combined release strategy, initial rapid release followed by prolonged drug release is required to maintain stable plasma concentration. Bimodal release tablets show an initial rapid drug release, followed by slow release of the drug substance, then a third phase of rapid drug release, i.e., tablets exhibit sigmoidal release profiles [11, 13–15].

5. Manufacturing technology

In the past decades, layered tablets have been gaining attention, thus increasing the requirement for the development of newer formulation techniques and technologies. However, most of the techniques are the same as that of a conventional tablet, some variations in compression are necessary. It is important to analyze physio-chemical properties, cohesive properties, compression, and compaction profiles of all the layers used individually before the production of layered tablets. The ultimate objective is to produce stable layered tablets, that remain in a single unit, without layer separation and reduce the bulk of the tablet [5, 16, 17].

5.1 OROS® push-pull technology

The system comprises two or more layers in which one or more layers contain active ingredients and others are push layers (**Figure 2**). The drug layer can be made of single or multi-components. Mostly poorly soluble drugs are incorporated. The drug release can be aided by the addition of suspending or osmotic agent. The tablet core can be surrounded by a semi-permeable membrane.

5.2 L-OROS tm Technology

This is used in the case of poorly soluble and insoluble drugs. By this technique a lipid soft gel product which holds the drug in a dissolved state is initially produced, then it is coated with a barrier membrane followed by an osmotic push layer and semipermeable membrane, as shown in **Figure 3**. An exit orifice is drilled at the end.

5.3 EN SO TROL technology

It is an integrated method to deliver the drug to enhance solubility and incorporate enhancers to achieve controlled drug release from the dosage form. A wicking agent is generally used.

6. DUREDAS™ technology

It is a dual drug delivery form consisting of two layers where one provides immediate release and sustained release of the same drug (**Figure 4**). An immediate-release layer is composed of granules with a matrix layer for the modified release of the drug. One or more hydrophilic polymers are used in such cases.

6.1 RoTab bilayer compression

It is one of the dynamic and widely trusted equipments used in compression on mono and bilayer tablets. It comes with software, which makes it easy to use. Due

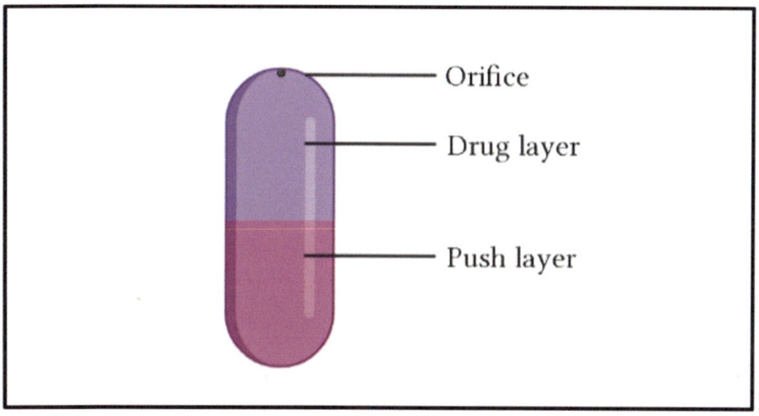

Figure 2.
Bilayer OROS push pull technology.

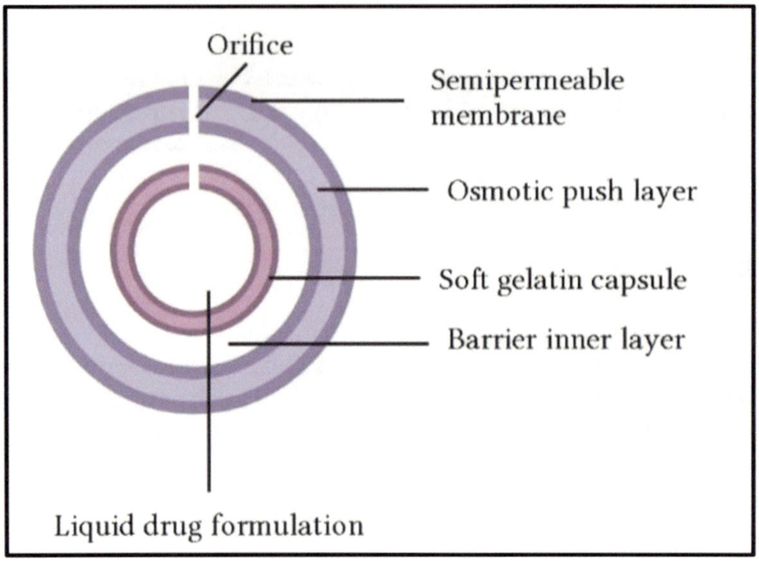

Figure 3.
L-OROS tm technology.

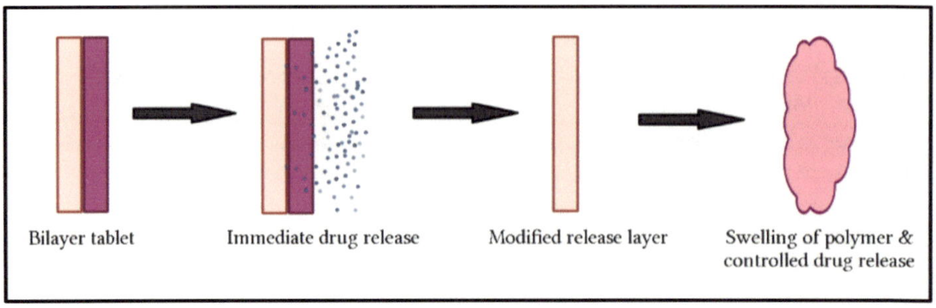

Figure 4.
Dual drug delivery dosage form.

to various controllable parameters and flexibility, it is of greater utility in R&D. Switching between mono and bilayer makes an impact on its desirability.

7. Challenges in manufacturing layered tablets

Apart from the common tableting problems, there are several other challenges that are more dominant in the case of layered tablets.

7. 1 Weight variation, sequence

Weight variation is generally studied in the case of solid unit dosage forms. The weight variation can be subjected to variation between units and also between the layers. Each layer should possess the predetermined weight without any major deviation in range. Individual layer weight [18]. It is preferable for the layers to have similar weight so that it aids produce required strength, weight distribution, appearance, and similar compression profiles.

7. 2 Mechanical strength

It is noted that excipients play important role in producing a high-quality layered tablet. Excipients that confer brittleness to the formulation are preferred to provide sufficient mechanical strength to layered tablets such that they can withstand mechanical pressure during production, packing, and transportation [19, 20].

7. 3 Lubrication

It is studied that increase in lubricant concentration, decreases the strength of interfacial bonding and can deteriorate the interfacial interaction between the layers [21, 22].

7. 4 Adhesion strength

The major challenge is holding the layers together which is dependent on interlayer adhesion strength between two or more layers used. In the production of layered tablets, initially, a central core is prepared by pre-compression, then the upper and lower layers are compressed around the central core. Necessary interlayer adhesion strength is required to hold these layers together as a single unit. Low compression force for the core and high compression force for layers can help in attaining adequate adhesion [23–25].

7. 5 Interlayer cross-contamination

There is a high possibility of cross-contamination between the adjacent layers. To overcome this, scraper plates are placed around the die fill to remove residual powder [26]. In some cases, suction and dust removers are also being used.

7. 6 Long term integrity and storage

The layered tablets should display a long-term physical and chemical integrity throughout the shelf life of the dosage form [28]. Temperature and humidity changes during storage have a greater impact on interlayer adhesion [27, 28].

7. 7 Size of the tablet

Attention has to be given to the size of the tablet, as multiple layers can lead to an increase in size, making it difficult to swallow. This can be handled by minimizing the separation layers. It is difficult to accommodate two drugs in high doses.

8. Evaluation of layered tablets

Most of the pre and post-compression evaluations are the same as that of a conventional tablet.

8.1 Pre-compression evaluations

Before the compression, the API and other excipients are evaluated to study the powder characteristics and micromeritics. The powder particle size is determined using a laser diffractometer. Various other powder properties like Hausner's ratio, Carr's index, and angle of repose are also determined before manufacturing a tablet. The moisture content of the powders is evaluated thermogravimetrically.

8.2 Post compression evaluations

8.2.1 Weight uniformity

The formulation should have a uniform weight within the batch. It is a major quality control test in the formulation of tablets. It is necessary to ensure that all tablets have weights within the tolerated limits to ensure intra and inter-batch uniformity data. About 20 tablets from each batch are evaluated for weight uniformity by determining individual weights.

8.2.2 Thickness

One serious drawback of layered tablets is the increased thickness. It should possess sufficient thickness to accommodate multiple layers of drug and inert materials. It should also be ensured that it lies within the swallowable limits. The thickness of the tablet is determined by the vernier caliper. It ensures that the tablet lies within the desired range, enabling easy swallowing.

8.2.3 Friability and hardness

To test tablets to withstand mechanical damage during processing, transport, and storage, friability and hardness are evaluated. About 10 tablets are weighed and loaded into the rotating drum of friability apparatus set at 100 rotations. Then the tablets are reweighed to calculate the weight lost. Hardness is the measure of the maximum pressure that a tablet can withstand. It is measured using instruments like Pfizer/Monsanto hardness tester.

8.2.4 Content uniformity

In order to assure that each tablet contains a labeled amount of API, they are evaluated using UV Visible spectrophotometer. Tablets are dissolved in suitable solvents and evaluated under a specific wavelength. In the case of more than one API, the simultaneous equation method is generally used.

8.2.5 Disintegration time

Time taken for a tablet to break down directly confers to the absorption. Faster disintegration promotes faster dissolution and absorption. The disintegration apparatus consists of disintegration vessels made up of mesh, immersed in a disintegration medium, which moves at specified cycles at the rate of 28-32 strokes per minute. The disintegration time is calculated as the time at which the tablet completely disintegrates.

8.2.6 In-vitro drug release

It is determined using dissolution apparatus to study the release profile and dissolution profile of the tablets. It directly influences the rate of absorption. Since it possesses more than one API, the simultaneous equation method is used to calculate the drug concentration in the sample by UV Visible spectrophotometer [29]. Tablets are dropped into the dissolution medium of 900 ml volume, maintained at 37 ± 0.5 °C. Based on the requirement Type I or II dissolution apparatus is selected. The paddle/basket is rotated at 25-100 rpm. Samples are withdrawn at a specific time period and evaluated UV spectroscopically.

8.2.7 Drug release kinetic

It is necessary to evaluate the kinetics of drug release as multiple layers may exhibit various release rates, which can confer to its profile. Each layer may exhibit a different release rate, characterizing sustain release and immediate release pattern is necessary.

8.2.8 Stability studies

It is one such star test common for all pharmaceutical products. Here stability of all the layers is studied. Layers may display different degrees of degradation. Shelf life is determined based on each layer's characteristics.

8.2.9 Morphology analysis

Physical qualities can be examined by visualization. The morphology of layered tablets can be visualized by Scanning Electron Microscopy using cross-section samples [30].

8.2.10 Thermal analysis

Thermal analysis is of greater interest in detecting drug-excipient, drug-drug, and excipient-excipient interactions in the formulation. Using Differential Scanning Calorimetry, molecular dispersion of drug substance in tablet matrix system can be identified [30].

8.2.11 Crystallinity

The crystalline and amorphous nature of drugs has a direct influence on their stability, solubility, and various other Physico-chemical properties. The crystal nature of drug substances in various layers is evaluated by using X-Ray Diffractometer (XRD). Possible transformation of drug nature from crystalline to amorphous form or vice versa during processing or storage can be studied [31].

9. Conclusion

The oral dosage form has gained its prominent position at the top of the chain. Even after decades of advancements and novel drug delivery approaches, oral tablets make up most of the pharmaceutics. Oral tablets are not only popular but also are most stable with a high degree of patient compliance. Speaking about enhancing oral tablets, layered tablets are an add-on. By weighing several parameters, layered tablets can be a vital approach in oral solid dosage forms. The layered tablets are gaining a lot of attention. Devising oral tablets using multiple layers makes it convenient over delivering multiple tablets. It enhances compliance and also offers a low capital investment and cost-effective production. From the perspective of manufacturers, clinicians, and patients, layered tablets remain preferable. Thus, greater focus can be shown on such technology in the future to explore more in this dosage form.

Acknowledgements

The authors are thankful to KMCH College of Pharmacy, Coimbatore, for their constant support.

Conflict of interest

The authors declare no conflict of interest.

Author details

Muthukumar Subramanian*, Chellam Sankar, Gayathri Rajaram and Vinesha Ravi
Department of Pharmaceutics, KMCH College of Pharmacy,
Coimbatore, Tamil Nadu, India

*Address all correspondence to: pharmmuthu@gmail.com

References

[1] Schenk M, Mueller C. The mucosal immune system at the gastrointestinal barrier. Best Practice & Research Clinical Gastroenterology. 2008;**22**:391-409

[2] Ensign LM, Cone R, Hanes J. Oral drug delivery with polymeric nanoparticles: The gastrointestinal mucus barriers. Advanced Drug Delivery Reviews. 2012;**64**:557-570

[3] Varum FJO, Mcconnell EL, Sousa JJS, Veiga F, Basit AW. Mucoadhesion and the gastrointestinal tract. Critical Reviews in Therapeutic Drug Carrier Systems. 2008;**25**:207-258

[4] Rathod RT, Misra D. FDC of montelukast with levocetirizine: Focus on bilayer technology. Journal of the Indian Medical Association. 2009;**107**:562-574

[5] Namrata M et al. A review on Bi-layer tablets. International Journal of Pharmaceutical and Phytopharmacological Research. 2013;**2**(4):240-246

[6] Serebruany VL, Malinin AI, Sane DC, Jilma B, Takserman A, Atar D, et al. Aggrenox and aspirin in patients after ischemic stroke: The Aggrenox versus aspirin therapy evaluation trial. European Journal of Pharmacology. 2004;**3**:315-324

[7] Efentakis M, Peponaki C. Formulation study and evaluation of matrix and three-layer tablet sustained drug delivery systems based on carbopols with isosorbite mononitrate. AAPS PharmSciTech. 2008;**9**:917-923

[8] Vimovo™: (naproxen/esomeprazole magnesium) delayed-release tablets. P T. 2010;**35**(9 Section 2):2-4

[9] Krishnaiah YSR, Karthikeyan RS, Gouri Sankar V, Satyanarayana V. Three-layer guar gum matrix tablet formulations for oral controlled delivery of highly soluble trimetazidine dihydrochloride. Journal of Controlled Release. 2002;**81**:45-56

[10] Charman SA, Charman WN. Oral modified-release delivery systems. In: Rathbone MJ, Hadgraft J, Roberts MS, editors. Modified-Release Drug Delivery Technology. London: Informa Healthcare; 2002. pp. 1-19

[11] Qiu Y, Chidambaram N, Flood K. Design, and evaluation of layered diffusional matrices for zero-order sustained-release. Journal of Controlled Release. 1998;**51**:123-130

[12] Gavate NT, Gondkar SB, Saundaga RS. Multilayer tablet: A new trend in solid dosage forms. World Journal of Pharmaceutical Sciences. 2013;**2**:271-284

[13] Yadav G, Bansak M, Thakur N, Khare SP. Multilayer tablets and their drug release kinetic models for oral controlled drug delivery system. Middle-East Journal of Scientific Research. 2013;**16**:782-795

[14] Maroni A, Zema L, Carea M, Sangalli ME. Oral pulsatile drug delivery systems. Expert Opinion on Drug Delivery. 2005;**2**:855-871

[15] More S, Ghodekar S, Rane B, Bavaskar K, Patil M, Jain A. Multilayered tablet: A novel approach for oral drug delivery. International Journal of Pharmaceutical Sciences and Research. 2015;**9**:872-882

[16] RoTab Bilayer Compression [Internet source]. Available from: www.durect.com. [Accessed: August 12, 2021]

[17] RoTab Bilayer Compression [Internet source]. Available from: www.port/technology.com. [Accessed: August 12, 2021]

[18] RoTab Bilayer Compression [Internet source]. Available from: https://www.mgamerica.com/equipment/rotab-bi-layer-tablet-press-for-bi-layer-tablets/. [Accessed: September 12, 2021]

[19] Van Veen B, Maarschalk KVDV, Bolhuis GK, Zuurman K, Frijlink HW. Tensile strength of tablets containing two materials with a different compaction behaviour. International Journal of Pharmaceutics. 2000;**203**:71-79

[20] Abdul S, Poddar SS. A flexible technology for modified release of drugs: Multi-layered tablets. Journal of Controlled Release. 2004;**97**:393-405

[21] Kottala N, Abebe A, Sprockel O, Bergum J, Nikfar F, Cuitino A. Evaluation of the performance characteristics of bilayer tablets: Part I. impact of material properties and process parameters on the strength of bilayer tablets. AAPS PharmSciTech. 2012;**13**:1236-1242

[22] Sugisawa K, Kaneko T, Sago T, Sato T. Rapid quantitative analysis of magnesium stearate in pharmaceutical powders and solid dosage forms by atomic absorption: Method development and application in product manufacturing. Journal of Pharmaceutical and Biomedical Analysis. 2009;**49**:858-861

[23] Cremer K, Asmussen B. Novel controlled-release tablet with erodible layers. Proceedings of the International Symposium on Controlled Release of Bioactive Materials. 1995;**22**:732-733

[24] Abdul S, Poddar SS. A flexible technology for modified release of drugs: multi-layered tablets. Journal of Controlled Release. 2004;**97**:393-405

[25] Desai D, Wang J, Wen H, Li X, Timmins P. Formulation design, challenges, and development considerations for fixed dose combination (FDC) of oral solid dosage forms. Pharmaceutical Development and Technology. 2013;**18**:1265-1276

[26] Park CR, Munday DL. Development and evaluation of a biphasic buccal adhesive tablet for nicotine replacement therapy. International Journal of Pharmaceutics. 2002;**237**:215-226

[27] Abebe A, Akseli I, Sprockel O, Kottala N, Cuitino AM. Review of bilayer tablet technology. International Journal of Pharmaceutics. 2014;**461**:549-558

[28] Kottala N, Abebe A, Sprockel O, Bergum J, Nikfar F, Cuitino A. Evaluation of the performance characteristics of bilayer tablets: part I. Impact of material properties and process parameters on the strength of bilayer tablets. AAPS PharmSciTech. 2012;**13**:1236-1242

[29] Kumar GH, Jaganathan K, Kumar RS, Peruma P. Formulation and in-vitro evaluation of bilayer floating tablets of Metformin hydrochloride and Sitagliptin phosphate. International Journal of Advanced Pharmaceutics. 2012;**2**(2):64-81

[30] Agiba AM, Abdel-Hamid S, Nasr M, Geneidi AS. Geriatric oriented high dose nutraceutical ODTs: Formulation and physicomechanical characterization. Curr Drug Delivery. 2018;**15**:267-277

[31] Agiba AM. Liquisolid technology: A state-of-the-art review on the current state, challenges, new and emerging technologies for next generation. Current Drug Delivery. 2020;**17**:736-754

Chapter 2

Orally Disintegrating Tablets

Fikadu Ejeta

Abstract

Research and development costs for a single new pharmaceutical that is introduced to the market are estimated to cost between $1 billion and $2 billion. Due to the high cost of development and the need to quickly access various technologies, it is more cost-effective (clinically and financially) to enhance current pharmaceuticals for potency, selectivity, drug metabolism, and dosing convenience before they reach the market. Orally dissolving tablets have been developed as a result. Pharmaceutical companies have created oral disintegrating tablets that dissolve or disintegrate in the mouth within a few seconds of being placed there in order to maximize the safety and efficacy of the medicine molecule. Because patients with weak physiological (patients with mental illnesses) and physical capacities can easily administer it to geriatrics, children, and patients with these conditions (patients suffering from dysphagia), as well as traveling patients who may not have easy access to water and where swallowing conventional solid oral-dosage forms presents difficulties, it has grown in popularity among a wide population. These tablets can be prepared in many ways like direct compression, freeze drying, sublimation, molding, and spray drying by using single or combinations of superdisintegrants or subliming agents.

Keywords: formulations, orally disintegrating tablets, immediate release, stability studies, pharmacokinetics, superdisintegrants

1. Introduction

To maximize the safety and effectiveness of the medication molecule, pharmaceutical companies have developed oral disintegrating tablets that dissolve or disintegrate in the mouth after a few seconds of being placed there. It has gained popularity among a large population because it can be administered with ease to patients with weak physiological (patients with mental illnesses) and physical capacities, geriatrics, children, and patients with these conditions (patients suffering from dysphagia), as well as traveling patients who might not have easy access to water and where swallowing conventional solid oral-dosage forms presents difficulties [1, 2].

The European Pharmacopoeia states that Orally Disintegrating Tablets (ODTs) are uncoated tablets that are intended to be placed in the mouth and then dispersed rapidly before being swallowed. The European Pharmacopeia specifies a limit of 3 minutes for the in vitro disintegration in water. A fast-dissolving drug delivery system is a novel drug delivery system that aims to improve the safety and efficacy of the drug molecule by formulating a dosage form that quickly dissolves in the mouth [3, 4]. Because it may be provided with ease to elderly patients, children, people with mental illness, people who have trouble swallowing, people who are traveling, and people who might not have access to water at all; it has gained popularity among the general population [5].

Liquid formulations for routinely used pediatric drugs, as well as for patients in an acute setting or with adherence issues, have been created by manufacturers. They are not without flaws, are frequently unstable, and have short shelf lives. Accurate dosage measurement and administration are also a challenge [6, 7]. As a result, both the pharmaceutical business and academics have recently become interested in the development of orally disintegrating tablets. Actually, ODTs are becoming more and more popular among patients, particularly those who are young and old and wish to have access to their prescriptions whenever they need it. Patients value these drugs' discretion and ease of use because they can be taken without water and start working right away [8]. As long as dispersion is rapid, bioavailability of the drug can be significantly greater than those observed from conventional tablet dosage forms [9].

1.1 Pharmacokinetic and pharmacodynamics consideration

As drug dissolves in saliva, it bypasses enterohepatic circulation and prevents first-pass metabolism by undergoing pre-gastric absorption. This improves bioavailability of the drug and reduces dosing frequency and dose-related untoward effects [10]. Orally disintegrating formulations are bioequivalent to the typical capsules now in use, with the added benefit of not requiring liquids. This allows for the management of emergent pain as soon as possible, regardless of the location or situation in which it occurs. The safety evaluation revealed that both orally disintegrating tablets and capsules were well tolerated, with no reported side effects. The similar maximum plasma concentrations (Cmax) achieved by both preparations are consistent with the lack of changes in safety parameters between the two formulations. Finally, from a practical standpoint, the availability of a bioequivalent tablet that can be eaten without liquids adds value because emergent pain can be addressed right away, regardless of where it occurs. This type of galenic formulation may also be beneficial for people who have difficulty swallowing or who have restricted mobility. It may also be of interest to institutionalized patients, as caregivers' jobs are made easier.

For example, salbutamol sulfate exhibits site-specific absorption in the stomach and upper parts of the small intestine [11]. Drug absorption requires molecules to be in solution at the absorption site. Conventional tablets may pass through the absorption site until they disintegrate and dissolve, resulting in reduced bioavailability. Because they appear as a solution at the absorption site, orally disintegrating tablets may increase the chances of being absorbed [12]. This may improve drug bioavailability, particularly for medicines with limited absorption sites in the small intestine [11, 13, 14].

Although albuterol and other ß2 agonists were formerly provided orally to provide a longer duration of action, this strategy is being phased out in favor of ß2 agonists that have a longer duration of action when administered via inhalation. Short-acting bronchodilators are the first line of treatment for COPD patients who have symptoms that come and go [15]. Drugs with very short half-lives need to be given at frequent dosing intervals to maintain therapeutic efficacy [16]. When the drug concentration is high and the enzyme is subjected to first-pass hepatic biotransformation [17], saturation occurs. As a result, the rate procedure is reduced to zero orders. As all of the enzyme molecules become complex with the drug, bioavailability may improve, and free drug may escape metabolism [11]. Drug bioavailability may be enhanced through oral cavity absorption as well as pregastric absorption of saliva-containing dispersed medicines that move down into the stomach. Furthermore, when compared to traditional tablets, the amount of medication susceptible to first-pass metabolism is reduced [5].

2. Formulations of orally disintegrating tablets

ODTs are frequently prepared for immediate release, but they can also be formulated for prolonged or controlled release. Rapid disintegration is an ODT feature as a result, during formulation at least one superdisintegrant is needed. But some scholars have used combinations of different superdisintegrants like crospovidone and starch glycolate [18], combinations of superdisintegrants, and subliming agents like ammonium bicarbonate [19].

Crospovidone is a water-insoluble tablet disintegrant and dissolution agent used at 2–8% concentration in tablets prepared by direct-compression methods [20]. This may vary depending on methods of manufacturing, types of excipients, and nature of active ingredients under investigation [21]. The superior disintegrant capability of crospovidone can be attributed to its rapid capillary action, faster hydration rate, and little tendency of gel formation. Crospovidone's high and rapid water absorption ability has a negative influence on wetting time. Due to its porous particle shape, it causes enormous wicking forces, further expanding and dissolving the tablet into finer particles. Crospovidone increased the crushing strength of tablets in a synergistic manner. This is due to its plastic character and binding capability, in addition to being an efficient disintegration agent; it acts as a highly compressible material in the dry state, hence increasing its concentration from 2–8% considerably enhanced the crushing strength of tablets. Ammonium bicarbonate is chemically inert and when subjected to high temperature and pressure, sublime due to its volatile nature resulting in highly porous structure in the tablets. It is utilized as a porosity-forming agent in tablets at a concentration of 2.5–20%. The solid, crystalline nature of ammonium bicarbonate accounts for its superiority. After sublimation, the leftover fractions of liquid volatile components in tablets solidify and serve as binders, but ammonium bicarbonate in residual concentration does not undergo this transformation and does not alter the mechanical characteristics of tablets [22, 23].

Excipient compatibility is responsible for mechanical strength, while high porosity is the key factor controlling quick disintegration of ODTs. Binder/disintegrant systems with dual benefits have solved both objectives in part. Mannitol has nice flavor and sweetening properties. Microcrystalline cellulose, on the other hand, has better mechanical characteristics for ODTs than mannitol. More than only good binding qualities in an excipient is required for the production of orally disintegrating tablets [24]. Amalgamation of cellulose and polyol-based excipients such as mannitol provides us with a clear criterion for developing directly compressed ODTs [23, 25]. The hardness of ODT is usually preferable between 4 and 8 kg in order to withstand handling during manufacturing, packaging, and transportation [26]. The hardness of tablets depends on the amount and types of binding agent present [27]. Therefore the change in hardness values of different ODTs observed in different amount and type of binding agents [28]. The hardness values for all tested tablets increase as the Microcrystalline cellulose to Mannitol ratio increases [23]. Occasionally sweetening agents like Aspartame (artificial sweetener) noncarcinogenic and can be consumed by diabetes patients, and; flavoring agents like vanillin can be used to mask unpleasant tastes and flavors of the active ingredients even though these are weak in taste masking. Much more intense sweeteners compared with sucrose with acceptable daily intake of 50 mg/kg. Vanilla flavor is a natural flavor that supplements and complements the sweetening agent [29]. There are many taste-masking techniques that have been reported in addition to adding flavors and sweeteners, coating drug particles with inert agents [30], inclusion complexes [31], microencapsulation [32], solid dispersions [26], molecular complexes of drug with other chemicals and prodrug by using ion exchange resins [33].

3. Techniques for manufacturing of ODTs

The Orally disintegrating tablets could be prepared using various techniques such as direct compression, lyophilization, sublimation, tablet molding, and spray drying [34, 35].

3.1 Direct compression

Direct compression is a simple, cost-effective solution to produce robust tablets that retain the appropriate disintegration properties. It also provides better stability of active pharmaceutical ingredients, fast dissolution, simple validation, and low microbial contamination. Moreover, ODDTs manufactured via direct compression tend to have a much higher drug-loading capacity and the final mass of these ODTs easily exceeds that of other formulation techniques. On the other hand, tablets produced via direct compression have much higher physical resistance but take longer to disintegrate [36]. The basic principle of direct compression involves combining disintegrants, or effervescent agents, and hydrophilic ingredients. Superdisintegrants incorporated in optimum concentrations are often used to achieve rapid disintegration of ODDTs, as well as a good mouth feel [37]. Crospovidone is the disintegrants of choice for fastest disintegration, shortest wetting time, enhanced rate of drug dissolution, and robust tablets. This is because it swells without forming gels which can slow tablet disintegration or dissolution. But, other superdisintegrants form gels when fully hydrated, particularly when a high amount is used some formulations to achieve desired tablet disintegration or drug dissolution [38].

3.2 Freeze drying

Freeze drying (lyophilization) is a process of removing water from a substance at lower temperatures under controlled conditions through sublimation [36]. This method has the advantage of allowing pharmaceutical compounds to be processed at lower temperatures, reducing sensitivity to thermal impacts, and allowing the solid to be kept in a dry environment with fewer stability issues. Because the resulting structures are relatively porous, lyophilization yields products that disintegrate more quickly than other solid dosage forms. Furthermore, the freeze-drying procedure causes the bulking agents in a formulation to have a glassy amorphous structure, which improves their disintegration capabilities. This approach produces ODTs with low mechanical strength that requires special packaging [26].

3.3 Sublimation

This method entails adding volatile chemicals such as ammonium bicarbonate, urea, naphthalene, and camphor to the other tablet ingredients before compressing them to make ODTs. Sublimation removes the volatile material trapped within the compressed tablets, resulting in the creation of pores within the formulation [22, 23, 39]. A high porosity while used for the enhancing disintegration rate of ODTs is undesirable for tablet mechanical strength [40]. Because many ODTs are porous, if the processing parameters are not optimal, the tablets can become more friable, regardless of hardness adjustments. Co-processed excipients must be employed to make mechanically hard ODTs without sacrificing disintegration time [23, 41].

3.4 Spray drying

Spray drying offers a quick and affordable method for getting rid of solvents and creating highly porous, fine powders that dissolve quickly. Rapid evaporation of the processing solvent during spray drying might result in the production of very porous, fine powder. Rapidly disintegrating pills can be made by spray drying [42]. This method uses a particulate support matrix, which is made by spray drying an aqueous composition comprising the support matrix and other ingredients into a highly porous and fine powder. The active components are subsequently added and the pills are crushed [43]. Hydrolyzed and nonhydrolyzed gelatins are used as supporting agents, mannitol is used as a bulking agent, sodium starch glycolate or croscarmellose sodium is used as a disintegrating agent, and an acidic and/or alkali material (e.g., sodium bicarbonate) is used to improve disintegration and dissolution [44].

3.5 Molding

This method creates solid dispersions known as ODDTs. Molded tablets are mainly manufactured from soluble components such as xylitol, lactose, glucose, sorbitol, sucrose, and mannitol. The powder mixture is wet with a hydroalcoholic solvent before being molded into tablets at a lower pressure than traditional tablet compression. The solvent is subsequently removed by air drying. Compressed tablets are much more compact than molded tablets. Their porous nature facilitates dissolution [44]. Unfortunately, the mechanical strength of molded tablets is often low. Erosion and breaking of the molded tablets occur frequently during tablet handling and when blister pockets are opened, posing potential stability issues.

4. Compatibility studies of formulation ingredients

The presence of polymorphic solids, which have different chemical and physical properties with biopharmaceutical effects in the dissolution rates and/or bioavailability as well as added excipients interactions either physically or chemically would be expected.. Therefore the physical characterization of the solid state of a drug has become an extremely important area in pharmaceutics and has been the subject of many studies involving different analytical methods.

4.1 Fourier Transform infrared spectroscopy (FTIR)

Fourier transform infrared analysis will be performed to detect any changes in chemical constitution of the drug after combining it with the excipients. Fourier transform infrared analysis will be performed to detect any interaction between the drug and ammonium bicarbonate and crospovidone. The compatibility between the drug and excipients used in many formulations is being studied using Fourier transform infrared spectroscopy (FTIR) at room temperature. Samples of drug and excipients and physical mixtures of both are commonly grinded and mixed thoroughly with KBr. at a 1:5 sample/KBr ratio. The KBr discs were prepared by compressing the powders at a pressure of 5 T for 5 min in a hydraulic press. The scanning range was 400 to 4000 $cm^{-1}$and the resolution was 8 cm^{-1}.

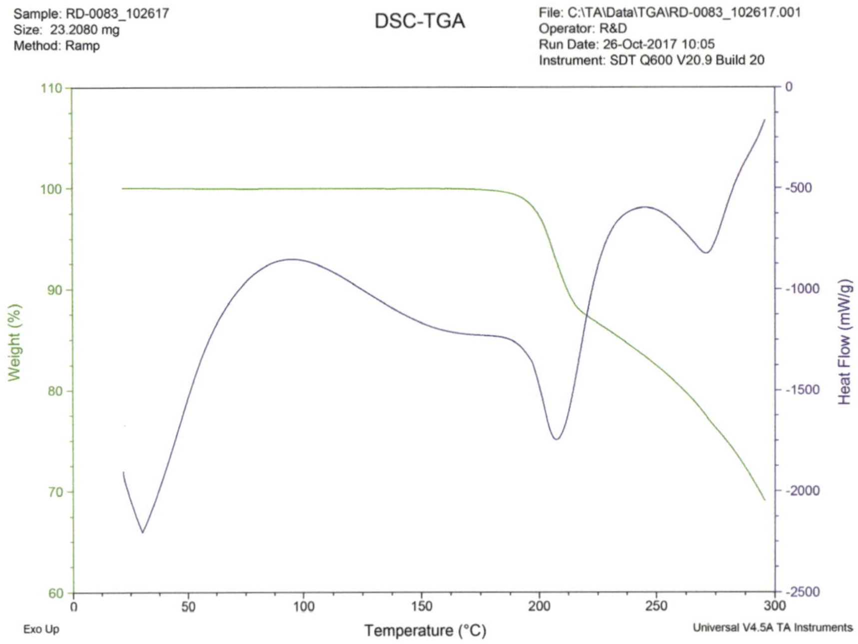

(A)

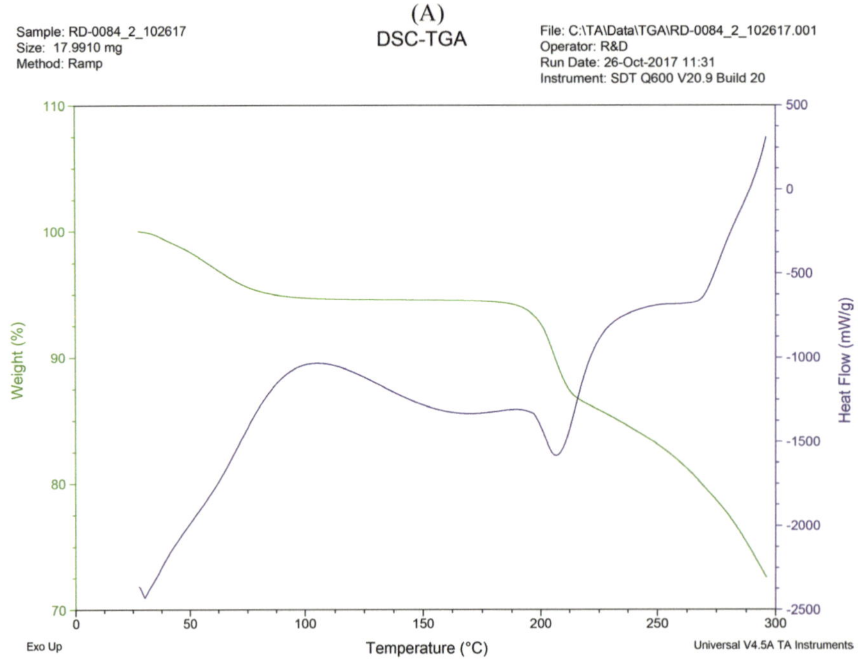

(B)

Figure 1.
The differential scanning calorimetric thermograms and thermogravimetric analysis of salbutamol (A) and salbutamol and crospovidone physical mixture (B).

4.2 Powder X-ray diffraction

X-ray powder diffraction (XRD) is a rapid analytical technique primarily used for phase identification of a crystalline material and is a unique method in determination of crystallinity of a compound. XRD will be performed to detect any crystallinity between the drug and ammonium bicarbonate and crospovidone. The powder X-ray diffraction patterns were measured using an X-ray diffractometer with Cu anode material. The diffraction pattern was measured with a voltage of 40kV and a current of 15 mA in the area of 0° <2Theta <100°.

4.3 Differential scanning calorimetry (DSC)

DSC is one of many types of thermal analysis techniques useful for characterizing pharmaceutical solids. Calorimetry is quite useful to measure chemical reactions such as cross-linking or curing reactions, oxidation processes, and thermal decomposition. Chemical reactions and the kinetics of these reactions under either inert or reactive atmospheres can be quantified nicely. DSC will be performed to detect any thermal decomposition between the drug and excipients. The thermal behavior can be estimated using differential scanning calorimetry by using Indium as a standard to calibrate the differential scanning calorimetry (DSC) temperature and enthalpy scale. The samples are hermetically sealed in aluminum pans and heated at a constant rate of 10°C/min, over a scanning temperature range of 0–400°C. An inert atmosphere was maintained by purging with nitrogen at a flow rate of 100 mL/min.

The DSC graphs of salbutamol sulfate and salbutamol sulfate and crospovidone physical mixture are presented in **Figure 1A** and **B**, respectively The DSC curve of the pure drug showed a sharp endothermic melting peak with the onset of about 210°C reaching maximum at 288°C. The DSC curve of salbutamol sulfate and crospovidone physical mixture showed a sharp endothermic melting peak with the onset of about 210°C reaching maximum at 283° C due to polymorphs (R) – salbutamol; as salbutamol sulfate exists in racemate forms S and R [45]. Besides, the small difference in the decomposition temperature could be associated with the different crystal morphology of the polymorphs [46, 47]. The thermogram of the corresponding physical mixture showed small endothermic peak indicating that amorphous form existed in the physical mixture which is in agreement with PXRD results. These might explain the faster dissolution of the drug in the physical mixture [26]. Thermogravimetric analysis (TGA) has been performed for the blends, and the weight loss due to the volatilization of the degradation products has been monitored as a function of temperature [48] as shown in **Figure 1A** and **B**, respectively [49]. Temperature at the maximum rate of weight loss (Tmax) improvement of salbutamol sulfate is ascribed to the compatibility of salbutamol sulfate and crospovidone in blends.

5. Stability studies of orally disintegrating tablets

The chemical and physical properties of the active substance and pharmaceutical excipients, the dosage form and its composition, the manufacturing process, the nature of the container-closure system, and the properties of the packaging materials are all factors that affect the stability of finished pharmaceutical products. In a stability study, the impact of changes in temperature, time, humidity, light intensity, and partial vapor pressure on the product in issue is evaluated. The effective or mean

Climatic area	Condition
Zone I Temperate	21°C/45% RH
Zone II Subtropical/mediterranean	25°C/60% RH
Zone III Hot/dry	30°C/35% RH
Zonev IVa Hot/humid	30°C/65% RH
Zone IVb Hot/very humid	30°C/75% RH

Table 1.
Long-term storage conditions area.

Study	Storage condition	
Long-term	25°C ± 2°C/60% RH ± 5% RH or 30°C ± 2°C/65% RH ± 5% RH or 30°C ± 2°C/75% RH ± 5% RH	12 months or 6 months
Intermediate	30°C ± 2°C/65% RH ± 5% RH	6 months
Accelerated	40°C ± 2°C/75% RH ± 5% RH	6 months

Table 2.
General storage conditions for pharmaceuticals.

kinetic temperature, rather than the recorded mean temperature, better depicts the actual situation; a product held for one month at 20°C and one month at 40°C will differ from one kept for two months at 30°C. Furthermore, storage circumstances are frequently such that the temperature is higher than the country's average climatic data would indicate as shown in **Tables 1** and **2** [50].

Long-term storage conditions are determined by the climatic condition under which the finished pharmaceutical products (FPP) is intended to be marketed.

Author details

Fikadu Ejeta
School of Pharmacy, College of Medicine and Health Sciences, Mizan-Tepi University, Ethiopia

*Address all correspondence to: fikaduejeta@gmail.com

References

[1] Katzung BG. Basic & Clinical Pharmacology. 10th ed. New York: McGraw-Hill; 2007. p. 579

[2] Aguilar JE, Montoya EG, Lozano PP, Negre JMS, Carmona MM, Grau JRT. New SeDeM-ODT expert system: An expert system for formulation of orodispersible tablets obtained by direct compression. In: JEBT-FT for PD A, editor. Formulation Tools for Pharmaceutical Development [Internet]. Philadelphia, USA: Woodhead Publishing; 2013. pp. 137-154. Available from: https://www.sciencedirect.com/science/article/pii/B9781907568992500062

[3] Koizumi KI, Watanabe Y, Morita K, Utoguchi N, Matsumoto M. New method of preparing high-porosity rapidly saliva soluble compressed tablets using mannitol with camphor, a subliming material. International Journal of Pharmaceutics. 1997;**152**(1):127-131

[4] Ibrahim MA, Abou El Ela AESF. Optimized furosemide taste masked orally disintegrating tablets. Saudi Pharmaceutical Journal. 2017;**25**(7):1055-1062. Available from: http://linkinghub.elsevier.com/retrieve/pii/S1319016417300671

[5] Tagarro I, Vauzelle-Kervroedan F, Díez MC. Pharmacokinetic assessment of a fast-release orodispersible tramadol tablet compared to a conventional tramadol capsule. Arzneimittel-Forschung/Drug Research. 2004;**54**(5):293-297

[6] Perioli L, D'Alba G, Pagano C. New oral solid dosage form for furosemide oral administration. European Journal of Pharmaceutics and Biopharmaceutics. 2012;**80**(3):621-629. DOI: 10.1016/j.ejpb.2011.12.011

[7] Singh J, Philip AK, Pathak K. Optimization studies on design and evaluation of orodispersible pediatric formulation of indomethacin. AAPS PharmSciTech. 2008;**9**(1):60-66. Available from: http://www.springerlink.com/index/10.1208/s12249-007-9018-4

[8] Abdelbary G, Prinderre P, Eouani C, Joachim J, Reynier JP, Piccerelle P. The preparation of orally disintegrating tablets using a hydrophilic waxy binder. International Journal of Pharmaceutics. 2004;**278**(2):423-433

[9] Martínez Terán ME, Flament MP. Development of multiparticulate orodispersible tablets for pediatric use. International Journal of Pharmaceutics. 2016;**511**(2):1143. DOI: 10.1016/j.ijpharm.2016.06.097

[10] Rahman Z, Siddiqui A, Khan MA. Orally disintegrating tablet of novel salt of antiepileptic drug: Formulation strategy and evaluation. European Journal of Pharmaceutics and Biopharmaceutics. 2013;**85**(**3**PART B):1300-1309. DOI: 10.1016/j.ejpb.2013.06.006

[11] Aarons L. Applied biopharmaceutics and pharmacokinetics. Journal of Clinical Pharmacy and Therapeutics. 1981;**6**(4):287-288

[12] Elder DP, Kuentz M, Holm R. Pharmaceutical excipients - quality, regulatory and biopharmaceutical considerations. European Journal of Pharmaceutical Sciences. 2016;**87**:88-99. DOI: 10.1016/j.ejps.2015.12.018

[13] García-Arieta A, Gordon J. On the BCS biowaivers of orally disintegrating

tablets. European Journal of Pharmaceutical Sciences. 2015;**66**:107-108

[14] Ono A, Sugano K. Application of the BCS biowaiver approach to assessing bioequivalence of orally disintegrating tablets with immediate release formulations. European Journal of Pharmaceutical Sciences. 2014;**64**:37-43. DOI: 10.1016/j.ejps.2014.08.003

[15] Somberg J. Pharmacotherapy: A pathophysiologic approach. American Journal of Therapeutics. 2007;**14**:418

[16] Zarmpi P, Flanagan T, Meehan E, Mann J, Fotaki N. Biopharmaceutical aspects and implications of excipient variability in drug product performance. European Journal of Pharmaceutics and Biopharmaceutics. 2017;**111**:1-15. DOI: 10.1016/j.ejpb.2016.11.004

[17] Nakpheng T, Songkarak S, Suwandecha T, Sritharadol R, Chunhachaichana C, Srichana T. Evidences for salbutamol metabolism by respiratory and liver cell lines. Drug Metabolism and Pharmacokinetics. 2017;**32**(2):127-134. Available from: http://www.sciencedirect.com/science/article/pii/S1347436716305493

[18] Pabari RM, Ramtoola Z. Effect of a disintegration mechanism on wetting, water absorption, and disintegration time of orodispersible tablets. Journal of Young Pharmacists. 2012;**4**(3):157-163. Available from: http://www.jyoungpharm.org/article/601

[19] Ejeta F, Gabriel T, Joseph NM, Belete A. Formulation, optimization and In vitro evaluation of fast disintegrating tablets of salbutamol sulphate using a combination of Superdisintegrant and subliming agent. Current Drug Delivery. 2022;**19**(1):129-141. Available from: https://www.eurekaselect.com/194046/article

[20] Moore I. Pharmaceutical excipients. In: Pharmazeutische Industrie [Internet]. Geneva, Switzerland: WHO; 2017. pp. 550-553. Available from: http://apps.who.int/prequal/trainingresources/pq_pres/workshop_China2010/english/22/002-Excipients.pdf

[21] Schiermeier S, Schmidt PC. Fast dispersible ibuprofen tablets. European Journal of Pharmaceutical Sciences. 2002;**15**(3):295-305

[22] Mishra SM, Rohera BD. An integrated, quality by design (QbD) approach for design, development and optimization of orally disintegrating tablet formulation of carbamazepine. Pharmaceutical Development and Technology. 2017;**22**(7):889-903. Available from: http://www.tandfonline.com/doi/full/10.1080/10837450.2016.1199566

[23] Ejeta F, Gabriel T, Joseph NM, Belete A. Formulation, optimization and in vitro evaluation of fast disintegrating tablets of salbutamol sulphate using a combination of Superdisintegrant and subliming agent [internet]. Current Drug Delivery. 2021;**19**:129-141. Available from: http://www.eurekaselect.com/node/194046/article

[24] Al-Khattawi A, Mohammed AR. Challenges and emerging solutions in the development of compressed orally disintegrating tablets. Expert Opinion on Drug Discovery. 2014;**9**(10):1109-1120. Available from: http://www.tandfonline.com/doi/abs/10.1517/17460441.2014.941802

[25] Al-Khattawi A, Koner J, Rue P, Kirby D, Perrie Y, Rajabi-Siahboomi A, et al. A pragmatic approach for engineering porous mannitol and mechanistic evaluation of particle performance. European Journal of Pharmaceutics and Biopharmaceutics.

2015;**94**:1-10. DOI: 10.1016/j.ejpb.2015.04.011

[26] Ahmed IS, Shamma RN, Shoukri RA. Development and optimization of lyophilized orally disintegrating tablets using factorial design. Pharmaceutical Development and Technology. 2013;**18**(4):935-943

[27] Chandrasekhar R, Hassan Z, AlHusban F, Smith AM, Mohammed AR. The role of formulation excipients in the development of lyophilised fast-disintegrating tablets. European Journal of Pharmaceutics and Biopharmaceutics. 2009;**72**(1):119-129. DOI: 10.1016/j.ejpb.2008.11.011

[28] Kaialy W, Khan U, Mawlud S. Influence of mannitol concentration on the physicochemical, mechanical and pharmaceutical properties of lyophilised mannitol. International Journal of Pharmaceutics. 2016;**510**(1):73-85. DOI: 10.1016/j.ijpharm.2016.05.052

[29] Walsh J, Cram A, Woertz K, Breitkreutz J, Winzenburg G, Turner R, et al. Playing hide and seek with poorly tasting paediatric medicines: Do not forget the excipients. Advanced Drug Delivery Reviews. 2014;**73**:14-33. DOI: 10.1016/j.addr.2014.02.012

[30] Ayenew Z, Puri V, Kumar L, Bansal A. Trends in pharmaceutical taste masking technologies: A patent review. Recent Patents on Drug Delivery & Formulation. 2009;**3**(1):26-39

[31] Arima H, Higashi T, Motoyama K. Improvement of the bitter taste of drugs by complexation with cyclodextrins: Applications, evaluations and mechanisms. Therapeutic Delivery. 2012;**3**(5):633-644

[32] Douroumis DD, Gryczke A, Schminke S. Development and evaluation of cetirizine HCl taste-masked oral disintegrating tablets. AAPS PharmSciTech. 2011;**2**(1):141-151. Available from: https://pubmed.ncbi.nlm.nih.gov/21181510

[33] Ge Z, Yang M, Wang Y, Shan L, Gao C. Preparation and evaluation of orally disintegrating tablets of taste masked phencynonate HCl using ion-exchange resin. Drug Development and Industrial Pharmacy. 2015;**41**(6):934-941. Available from: http://www.tandfonline.com/doi/full/10.3109/03639045.2014.914529

[34] Gad SCOX. Pharmaceutical Manufacturing Handbook. New Jersey: John Wiley & Sons; 2008

[35] Ghourichay MP, Kiaie SH, Nokhodchi A, Javadzadeh Y. Formulation and quality control of orally disintegrating tablets (ODTs): Recent advances and perspectives. BioMed Research International. 2021;**2021**:1-12

[36] Stoltenberg I, Breitkreutz J. Orally disintegrating mini-tablets (ODMTs) - a novel solid oral dosage form for paediatric use. European Journal of Pharmaceutics and Biopharmaceutics. 2011;**78**(3):462-469. DOI: 10.1016/j.ejpb.2011.02.005

[37] Bi YX, Sunada H, Yonezawa Y, Danjo K. Evaluation of rapidly disintegrating tablets prepared by a direct compression method. Drug Development and Industrial Pharmacy. 1999;**25**(5):571-581. Available from: http://www.tandfonline.com/doi/full/10.1081/DDC-100102211

[38] Mizumoto T, Masuda Y, Yamamoto T, Yonemochi E, Terada K. Formulation design of a novel fast-disintegrating tablet. International Journal of Pharmaceutics. 2005;**306**(1-2):83-90

[39] Oh TO, Kim JY, Ha JM, Chi SC, Rhee YS, Park CW, et al. Preparation of

highly porous gastroretentive metformin tablets using a sublimation method. European Journal of Pharmaceutics and Biopharmaceutics. 2013;**83**(3):460-467. DOI: 10.1016/j.ejpb.2012.11.009

[40] Fukami J, Yonemochi E, Yoshihashi Y, Terada K. Evaluation of rapidly disintegrating tablets containing glycine and carboxymethylcellulose. International Journal of Pharmaceutics. 2006;**310**(1-2):101-109

[41] Moqbel HA, ElMeshad AN, El-Nabarawi MA. A pharmaceutical study on chlorzoxazone orodispersible tablets: Formulation, in-vitro and in-vivo evaluation. Drug Delivery. 2016;**23**(8):2998-3007. Available from: https://www.tandfonline.com/doi/full/10.3109/10717544.2016.1138340

[42] Corrigan DO, Corrigan OI, Healy AM. Physicochemical and in vitro deposition properties of salbutamol sulphate/ipratropium bromide and salbutamol sulphate/excipient spray dried mixtures for use in dry powder inhalers. International Journal of Pharmaceutics. 2006;**322**(1-2):22-30

[43] King KR, Wang CCJ, Kaazempur-Mofrad MR, Vacanti JP, Borenstein JT. Biodegradable microfluids. Advanced Materials. 2004;**16**(22):2007-2012

[44] Jeong SH, Takaishi Y, Fu Y, Park K. Material properties for making fast dissolving tablets by a compression method. Journal of Materials Chemistry. 2008;**18**(30):3527-3535. Available from: http://xlink.rsc.org/?DOI=b800209f

[45] Palacio MA, Cuffini S, Badini R, Karlsson A, Palacios SM. Solid-state characterization of two polymorphic forms of R-albuterol sulfate. Journal of Pharmaceutical and Biomedical Analysis. 2007;**43**(4):1531-1534

[46] Chiou H, Li L, Hu T, Chan HK, Chen JF, Yun J. Production of salbutamol sulfate for inhalation by high-gravity controlled antisolvent precipitation. International Journal of Pharmaceutics. 2007;**331**(1):93-98

[47] Columbano A, Buckton G, Wikeley P. A study of the crystallisation of amorphous salbutamol sulphate using water vapour sorption and near infrared spectroscopy. International Journal of Pharmaceutics. 2002;**237**(1-2):171-178

[48] Ma X, Jiugao Y, Wang N. Compatibility characterization of poly(lactic acid)/ poly(propylene carbonate) blends. Journal of Polymer Science Part B: Polymer Physics. 2006;**44**(1):94-101

[49] Ejeta F. Recent formulation advances and preparation of orally disintegrating tablets. International Journal of Pharmaceutical Compounding. 2022;**26**(5):370-377

[50] WHO. Annex 5: Guidelines for stability testing of pharmaceutical products containing well established drug substances in conventional dosage forms. World Health Organization Technical Report Series. 1996;**863**:65-80. Available from: https://www.paho.org/hq/dmdocuments/2008/6_Annex_5_report_34.pdf

Chapter 3

Multifunctional Roles of PVP as a Versatile Biomaterial in Solid State

Marouene Bejaoui, Haykel Galai, Fathi Touati and Salah Kouass

Abstract

Polyvinylpyrrolidone (PVP) has proven to be a highly versatile material, as evidenced by its long history as multifunctional biomaterial with a wide range of high-performance applications (e.g., tissue engineering, drug delivery systems, and ophthalmologic applications). PVP was frequently used in medical and pharmaceutical field due to its several interesting properties (higher glass transition temperature, water solubility, biocompatibility, biodegradability, chemical stability, very good adhesive, and emulsifying agent). This chapter highlights the multifunctional roles of PVP in pharmaceutical formulations in solid state. In fact, PVP acted as a stabilizing agent for various amorphous drug molecules by minimizing their molecular mobility. Physical stabilization resulted from the reinforcement of intermolecular interactions in binary or ternary systems due to the synergetic effect of PVP. This made it possible to overcome several challenges for drug formulations (e.g., solubility and bioavailability weakness, physical instability under stress conditions, complexation efficiency of cyclodextrin molecules). In this chapter, the effect of PVP on the binary solid dispersion (indomethacin:kaolin) is discussed. We have shown that PVP enhanced physical stability of amorphous indomethacin under stress conditions (at RH: 75% and T = 40°C for three months), leading to the improvement of drug aqueous solubility by suppressing kaolin adsorption effect.

Keywords: biomaterial, PVP, molecular mobility, physical stability, water solubility, solid dispersion, kaolin, indomethacin

1. Introduction

Polyvinylpyrrolidone (PVP) is widely employed as a multifunctional material and it was approved by the US Food and Drug Administration as a safe polymer for biological experiments due to its simple processability, biocompatibility, and non-antigenicity [1, 2]. The biomedical and pharmaceutical fields are among the most explored (**Figure 1**). Recently, PVP is considered as the most promising polymers, not only for the development of new pharmaceutical formulations [3, 4] but also for the optimization of several properties of bioactive glasses [2, 5]. This chapter highlights the link between PVP and some bioactive glasses. The multifunctional roles of PVP in pharmaceutical field were also discussed, focusing on the effect of PVP in terms of physical stabilization and solubility enhancement of various drug formulations in solid state (milling method as example).

IntechOpen

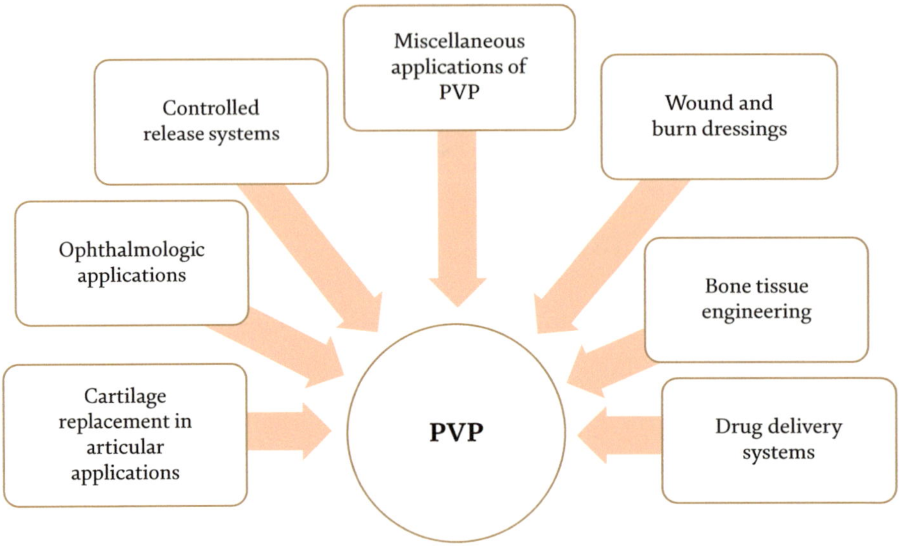

Figure 1.
Schematic representations of various PVP applications [2].

2. The usage of polyvinylpyrrolidone (PVP) in biomaterials

PVP was largely employed as a reinforcing material for biocomposites in a variety of applications, including bone tissue engineering, soft implants, biosensors, and artificial cartilage substitutes [2]. PVP can also be used in the fabrication of PVA hydrogels-based composite scaffolds for bone tissue engineering [6].

Cheng et al. have shown that, in the case of bioactive glass ceramics (BG), PVP induced faster apatite deposition and maintained the hybrid structure during electrospinning and pre-oxidation. This led to bioactivity improvement of bioactive glass [5]. For bioactive glass fibers (sol-gel synthesis), Hatcher [7] have demonstrated that PVP facilitated the synthesis process and the control of the rheological properties (more homogeneous fibrous material). PVP acted as a stabilizer by preventing gelation of the sample for 4 months. This was effective for enhancing *in vitro* bioactivity and increased proliferation of such bioactive glass fibers [7].

Moreover, Xia et al., have also shown that the addition of PVP resulted in sufficient chain entanglement and the formation of smooth bioactive glass nanofibers (electrospinning technique combined with sol-gel processing) [8]. Borate-modified bioactive glass [9] (burning-out method) was successfully achieved thanks to PVP, which greatly improved the blend's homogeneity. Ali et al. have obtained cerium-doped bioactive glass nanoparticles (scaffold fabrication) [10] by optimization of its mechanical properties using PVP. **Table 1** presents a list of published works focusing on bioactive glasses involving PVP.

Otherwise, PVP was used in some biomaterials for articular cartilage replacement because of its high hydrophilicity, which aids in the lubricating conditions of the resulting hydrogel [12]. PVP-based hydrogel was also obtained by radiation crosslinking and was effective for skin regeneration and wound dressing [13]. Multifunctional chitosan/PVP/45S5 Bioglass® scaffolds were also innovative for bone tissue engineering applications because of their outstanding bioactivity and *in situ* antibiotic-releasing capability [11]. PVP acted as stabilizer by inhibiting the enzymatic degradation of chitosan [11].

Bioactive glass	Authors
Bioactive glass-ceramics (BG)	Cheng et al. [5]
Bioactive glass fibers (sol-gel synthesis)	Hatcher [7]
Borate-modified bioactive glass (burning-out method)	Abdelghany et al. [9]
Cerium-doped bioactive glass nanoparticles (scaffold fabrication)	Ali et al. [10]
The 45S5 Bioglass® (BG)	Yao et al. [11]
Bioactive glass nanofibers (electrospinning technique combined with sol-gel processing)	Xia et al. [8]

Table 1.
List of published works on bioactive glasses involving PVP.

3. Multifunctional roles of PVP in pharmaceutical field

PVP (**Figure 2**) has several advantages in the pharmaceutical fields, and it acted as a stabilizer, a protective agent, a binder, a lubricating, a crystallization inhibitor, and a bioavailability enhancer for several active pharmaceutical ingredients (API) [4, 14]. It is widely known that PVP exhibited a higher solubility in water and polar solvents [15], and it also has a higher glass transition temperature (165 ± 1°C [16]) and was chemically stable in dry conditions [15]. Such physicochemical properties of PVP (**Table 2**) make it a versatile polymer with effective abilities in pharmaceutical field.

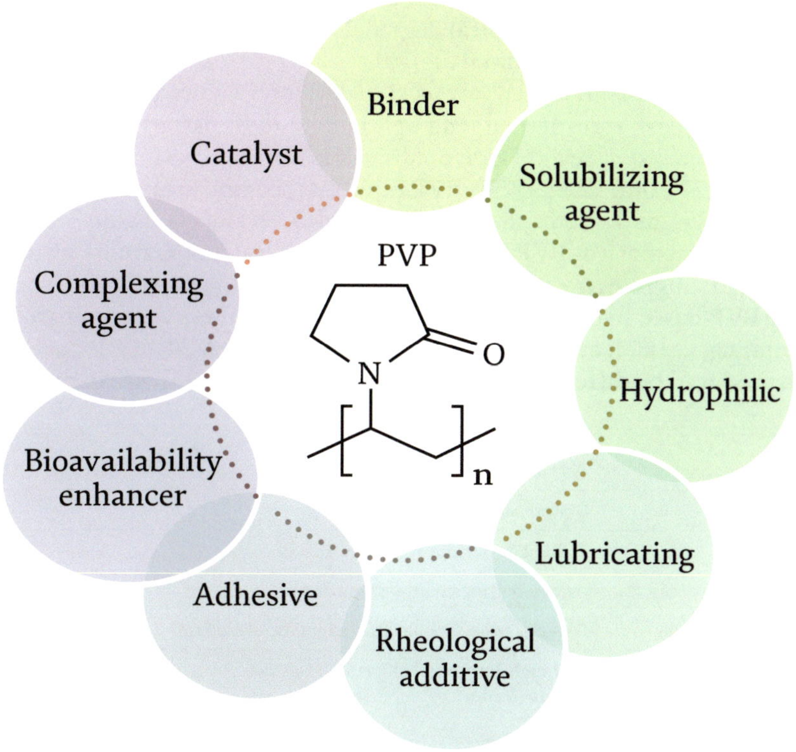

Figure 2.
Various pharmaceutical applications of PVP [14].

Properties	Details
Cas number	9003-39-8 [15]
Description	Hygroscopic amorphous white powder [15]
Formula	$(C_6\,H_9\,NO)_n$ [15]
Molecular weight	2500–30,00,000 D [15]
IUPAC name	l-ethenylpyirolidin-2-one [15]
Other names	Povidone, PVP, polyvidone, plasdone, Kollidon, poly [l-(2-oxo-pyrrolidinyl)ethylene], 1-vinyl-2-pyrroli-dinone polymer, 2-pyrrolidinone-l-ethenyl-homopolymer [15]
Solubility	Soluble in water, polar solvents, acids, and amines. Insoluble in ethers, hydrocarbons, mineral oil, and some esters [15]
Glass transition temperature	165 ± 1°C [16]
Stability	Chemically stable in dry form [15]
K value	Range 10–120 [15]

Table 2.
Physicochemical properties of PVP [15].

Many published works have shown the ability of PVP to enhance complexation, thus influencing drug solubility and stability [17]. Valero et al. have already shown that PVP enhanced the inclusion complex formation in the presence of β-cyclodextrin and naproxen molecules [18]. PVP has been proven to be an effective solubilizer for various β-cyclodextrin complexes [19]. Chemical stability can be also enhanced by PVP in solid state, and the chemical degradation of cilazapril was considerably inhibited by solid dispersion within PVP [20].

On the other hand, PVP was largely used to develop various drug delivery systems, including oral, topical, transdermal, and ophthalmic administration [2, 4, 19]. PVP-based fibers composed of several active substances were successfully achieved [21]. PVP hydrogels [22], oral tablets [23], PVP films [24], composite nanoparticles [25], microcapsules [26], and microspheres [27] were also developed. **Table 3** [3, 22, 24, 28–43] shows a summary of PVP-based drug delivery systems. Gamma irradiation, crosslinking, casting, electrospinning, and grafting were the most used techniques to produce PVP-based hydrogels [22, 31, 32]. PVP-based fibers were prepared by electrospinning, coaxial, and sequential electrospinning [33, 34]. PVP-based tablets were also produced by different techniques: 3D Printing [35, 36], spray drying or ball

Drug delivery systems	Active compound involved	Authors
Nanoparticles	Ciprofloxacin, paclitaxel, curcumin	[28–30]
Hydrogels	Salicylic acid, ketoprofen, amoxicillin	[22, 31, 32]
Fibers	Indomethacin, emodin, ibuprofen	[3, 33, 34]
Tablets (3D printing)	Dipyridamole, theophylline, pantoprazole sodium	[3, 35, 36]
Films	Fentanyl, ibuprofen haloperidol. Diltiazem hydrochloride & indomethacin	[24, 37–39]
Microparticles	Andrographolide, celecoxib, cefuroxime axetil, nimesulide	[40–43]

Table 3.
Examples of PVP-based drug delivery systems [3, 22, 24, 28–43].

milling followed by compression, direct or double compression, solvent evaporation or wet granulation followed by compression and supercritical impregnation [3]. Up to now, solution casting was frequently used to obtain PVP-based films [24, 37–39]. Drug-loaded PVP particles can be prepared by several techniques including spray drying, co-grinding, supercritical-assisted atomization (SAA), supercritical antisolvent (SAS) process, coacervation, freeze drying, and wet chemical method [40–42].

Regardless of preparation method, PVP-based solid dispersions were widely employed for several poorly soluble drug molecules in order to enhance their dissolution rate, for example, indomethacin (IND), sulfisoxazole, sulfathiazole, phenytoin, chloramphenicol, furosemide, tadalafil, nifedipine, naproxen, carbamazepine, ibuprofen, celecoxib, silymarin, nimodipine, β-lapachone, gliclazide, carvedilol [2, 4, 18, 19, 44–47]. Actually, solid dispersion technology by milling is one of the most attractive techniques for PVP-drug formulations [48]. Such technique was considered as environmental, scalable, economic, and simpler than other conventional methods [49]. In fact, solubility enhancement and physical stability of amorphous ibuprofen (at RH: 75%/T = 40°C for 6 months) can be achieved by ternary system formation (ibuprofen/β-cyclodextrin/PVP K30) in the ratio (1:1:0.5 w/w) [50]. This led to a 1.5–2-fold increase in the ibuprofen dissolution rate only after 10 min [50]. Such system was obtained by milling the drug in solid state at room temperature (25°C). PVP has undoubtedly reinforced synergy between compounds by establishing intermolecular H-bonds and electrostatic interactions between ibuprofen and β-cyclodextrin molecules [50]. Gupta et al. have shown that the antiplasticizing effect of PVP plays an important role in the stabilization of amorphous celecoxib (CLX) obtained by mechanical grinding, and this effect reduces the molecular mobility of the API and inhibits its recrystallization [51]. It has also been shown that ternary mixtures containing two excipients (PVP/MEG) have a greater CLX-solubilizing effect than that obtained by binary mixtures (PVP/CLX) [52]. Dissolution rate of bicalutamide was also enhanced by physical stabilization of its amorphous state using PVP [53].

Furthermore, several pharmaceutical products are formulated with PVP, for example, Betadine®, Inadine®, Prevail-FX®, ScrubCare®, and DuraPrep® [4]. Various studies have recently reported that PVP-iodine could be explored as a preventive aid against COVID-19 thanks to its antibacterial, antifungal, and antiviral properties [54].

3.1 The effect of PVP on indomethacin: kaolin solid dispersion

In our recent published work [55], we have studied the solid dispersion of binary system (indomethacin/kaolin) in the presence of PVP K30 by co-milling technique [55]. The milling procedure was carried out in a high-energy planetary ball mill (Pulverisette 7, Fritsch), using the stable γ form of indomethacin (IND, **Figure 3**). The milling parameters were optimized in order to avoid polymorphic transformations or chemical degradation of drug molecules [55].

Main results of characterization techniques are summarized in **Table 4** (curves not shown, [55]). According to XRD results [55], the addition of variable amount of PVP to the binary mixture (IND:kaolin, in 1:1 ratio) led to the loss of drug crystallinity. IND particles were totally coated by amorphous films of the polymer as shown by SEM micrographs (**Table 4**), and this was completely different to that observed in the binary mixture (IND:kaolin, in 1:1 ratio) [55]. Amorphous drug molecules maintain its physical stability even after exposure to stress conditions (RH: 75% and T = 40°C) for 6 months [55]. The stabilization of amorphous Indomethacin dispersed within kaolin was explained by different factors.

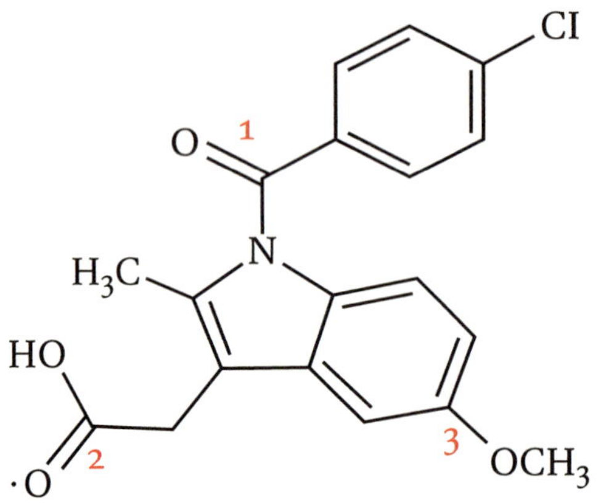

Figure 3.
Indomethacin molecule.

On the one hand, FTIR results have shown that C=O band (cyclic dimer) of IND shifted toward higher frequencies; however, the C=O (benzoyl) band shifted to lower frequencies and merged with the (C=O) band of PVP [55]. ^{13}C NMR spectroscopy has also indicated an upfield shift of IND carbon peak bound to methoxy groups and carbonyl group (2), which disappeared in the presence of 75% of PVP, while the C=O peak of PVP shifted toward higher values (from 176 ppm to 161 ppm) and merged with indomethacin peak [55]. The same behavior was already reported for IND: SiO_2 solid dispersion obtained by co-milling and this is due to intermolecular interactions between siloxane bonds and the oxygen of methoxy or carbonyl groups in IND molecules [56]. Therefore, FTIR and NMR results suggested the establishment of hydrogen bonds between carbonyl group of PVP and carboxylic group of indomethacin [55].

On the other hand, DSC curves have shown the appearance of a single transition event (Tg) that suggests the miscibility of the components in such mixture, and melting event of IND disappeared indicating complete conversion from crystalline to amorphous state [55]. The antiplasticizing effect of PVP has undoubtedly reduced the molecular mobility of amorphous drug molecules leading to its physical stability as shown by the XRD results [55].

According to previous results, the synergy of different factors could explain the stabilization of amorphous IND under stress conditions: hydrogen bonds formation between PVP and drug molecules, antiplasticizing effect of PVP, and hydrophilicity enhancement. This resulted in suppressed recrystallization of amorphous IND by inhibiting its molecular mobility [55].

In the case of binary mixtures (IND:kaolin), drug solubility decreased (**Table 5**) and this was attributed to kaolin adsorption effect [57]. Such attenuation occurred for many kaolin-based formulations [13], which constitutes an impediment for pharmaceutical use of kaolin [58]. As a result of PVP addition, water solubility of Indomethacin has been considerably improved (**Table 5**) in ternary systems [55]. By adding 75% of PVP to the binary system (in 1:1 ratio), water solubility increased about 4.5-folds [55].

It was already shown that PVP has a potential ability to enhance drug solubility, in many ternary systems [59]. Adding PVP to the binary solid dispersion (sodium lauryl sulfate/ibuprofen) was more efficacious in terms of drug dissolution enhancement [59]. Mahapatra et al. have shown that PVP has better enhanced valsartan solubility than β-cyclodextrin and hydroxypropyl β-cyclodextrin [60]. Dissolution rate enhancement

	DSC	XRD	RMN^{15}C	FTIR	SEM micrographs
BM	• A decrease of melting temperature T_f (IND)	• Partial disappearance of drug X-ray diffraction peaks	• No remarkable shifts	v(C=O)band (benzoyl) decreased	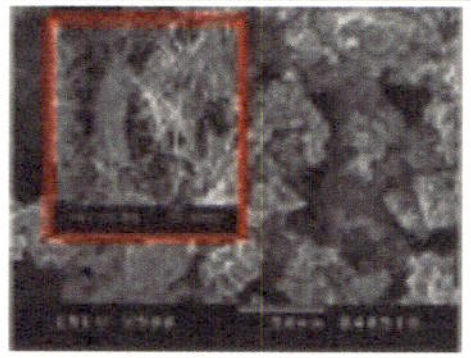 Apparition of amorphous microfibers adsorbed at the surface of kaolin [55]
TM	• Disappearance of drug melting event • Tg (IND) increased (Tg = 47 ± 1°C in the presence of 75% PVP)	• Appearance of halos and loss of drug crystallinity	• Upfield shift of IND carbon peaks (2 and 3) • Downfield shift of C=O peak of PVP	v (C=O)band (cyclic dimer) increased v (C=O)band (benzoyl) decreased	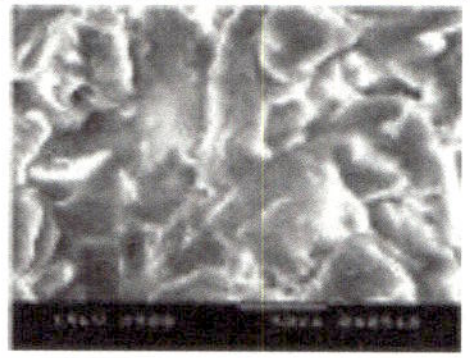 Drug particle was totally coated by amorphous films of the polymer [55]

Table 4.
Summary of characterization results for binary (BM) and ternary systems (TM) [55].

Samples	Solubility (µg/ml)
IND	9.33 ± 0.05
50% IND + 50% kaolin (BM)	8.38 ± 0.05
25% IND + 75% kaolin	6.01 ± 0.05
BM + 10% PVP	16.66 ± 0.1
BM + 25% PVP	29.05 ± 0.1
BM + 50% PVP	43.44 ± 0.1
BM + 75% PVP	44.44 ± 0.1

Table 5.
Water solubility measurement of indomethacin in binary (BM) and ternary systems [55].

of efavirenz was successfully obtained by ternary solid dispersion using PVP and polyethylene glycol 8000 [61]. In addition to aforesaid, we have recently reported that solubility enhancement of poorly soluble drugs can be achieved by co-milling the drug in the presence of multiple carriers, and this led to the formation of physically stable amorphous system and was more effective than simple binary systems [62].

4. Conclusion

In summary, the versatility of PVP comes from its multiple utilizations as multi-functional additive in biomedical and pharmaceutical fields. PVP has promoted the actual advances in bioactive glass design (optimizing mechanical properties, enhancing *in vitro* bioactivity, increasing proliferation and homogeneity of the material). The use of PVP in bone tissue engineering and scaffolds fabrication has grown considerably in recent years and constitutes a crucial element for designing new biomaterials. Pharmaceutical field has also profited from physicochemical properties of PVP that mainly acted as stabilizer, a crystallization inhibitor, and a solubility enhancer for several poorly soluble drugs in solid state. Solid dispersion in the presence of PVP was proven to be a potential strategy for improving drug solubility in binary and ternary systems. It has also enhanced complexation abilities for many β-cyclodextrin complexes in solid state. In this chapter, we have shown that PVP was able to overcome solubility challenge for indomethacin:kaolin solid dispersion by suppressing the adsorption effect of clay mineral and stabilizing amorphous drug molecules under stress conditions. Stabilization of amorphous drug formulations was correlated with the synergy of different PVP abilities: antiplasticizing effect, hydrogen bond formation between drug and carrier, and hydrophilicity enhancement. Thus, PVP can be considered as a promising material that may contribute to the development of new pharmaceutical products in order to face the current challenges in the medical field.

5. Perspectives

It is necessary to further investigate on the mechanisms and nature of interactions within bioactive glass materials containing PVP. More attention should be accorded to the role of PVP in drug formulations composed of clay minerals.

Acknowledgements

The authors thank Pr. Abdessalem Haj Amara (FSB, Tunisia) for his considerable inputs and helpful discussions. On the other hand, the authors confirmed that this research work did not receive any specific funding.

Conflict of interest

The authors declare that they have no conflict of interest.

Author details

Marouene Bejaoui*, Haykel Galai, Fathi Touati and Salah Kouass
LMTA, Institut National de Recherche et d'analyses Physico-Chimiques de Sidi-Thabet, Sidi Thabet, Tunisia

*Address all correspondence to: marouene2010@gmail.com

References

[1] Smith LE, Rimmer S, MacNeil S. Examination of the effects of poly (N-vinylpyrrolidinone) hydrogels in direct and indirect contact with cells. Biomaterials. 2006;**27**(14):2806-2812

[2] Teodorescu M, Bercea M, Morariu S. Biomaterials of PVA and PVP in medical and pharmaceutical applications: Perspectives and challenges. Biotechnology Advances. 2019;**37**(1): 109-131

[3] Franco P, De Marco I. The use of poly (N-vinyl pyrrolidone) in the delivery of drugs: A review. Polymers. 2020;**12**(5): 1114. DOI: 10.3390/polym12051114

[4] Kurakula M, Rao GK. Type of article: Review pharmaceutical assessment of polyvinylpyrrolidone (PVP): As excipient from conventional to controlled delivery systems with a spotlight on COVID-19 inhibition. Journal of Drug Delivery Science and Technology. 2020;**60**:102046. DOI: 10.1016/j.jddst.2020.102046

[5] Cheng D, Xie R, Tang T, Jia X, Cai Q, Yang X. Regulating micro-structure and biomineralization of electrospun PVP-based hybridized carbon nanofibers containing bioglass nanoparticles via aging time. RSC Advances. 2016;**6**(5):3870-3881. DOI: 10.1039/C5RA23337B

[6] Nkhwa S, Lauriaga KF, Kemal E, Deb S. Poly(vinyl alcohol): Physical approaches to designing biomaterials for biomedical applications. In: Conference Papers in Science. Vol. 2014. Hindawi: Publishing Corporation; 2014. DOI: 10.1155/2014/403472

[7] Hatcher BM. Polyvinylpyrrolidone modified bioactive glass fibers as tissue constructs: Synthesis, characterization, and rat mesenchymal stem cell response [Doctoral dissertation]. USA: University of Florida; 2002

[8] Xia W, Zhang D, Chang J. Fabrication and in vitro biomineralization of bioactive glass (BG) nanofibres. Nanotechnology. 2007;**18**(13):135601. DOI: 10.1088/0957-4484/18/13/135601

[9] Abdelghany AM, Meikhail MS, Hegazy E, Badr SI, Agag DA. Synthesis of borate modified bioactive glass scaffold using PVP burning-out method for bone tissue replacement. Biointerface Research in Applied Chemistry. 2019;**9**:4044-4049. DOI: 10.33263/BRIAC94.044049

[10] Ali A, Ekram B, El-Deen LS, Elkholy MM, Abd BM, Hady E. Preparation and investigation of novel porous scaffolds containing hydroxyethyl cellulose/poly vinyl pyrrolidone/cerium doped bioactive glass nanoparticles. International Journal of Latest Transactions in Engineering and Science. 2019;**8**(2):1-6

[11] Ma R, Xiong D, Miao F, Zhang J, Peng Y. Friction properties of novel PVP/PVA blend hydrogels as artificial cartilage. Journal of Biomedical Materials Research Part A: An Official Journal of The Society for Biomaterials, The Japanese Society for Biomaterials, and The Australian Society for Biomaterials and the Korean Society for Biomaterials. 2010;**93**(3):1016-1019

[12] Hu Y, Yan P, Fu L, Zheng Y, Kong W, Wu H, et al. Polyvinyl alcohol/polyvinyl pyrrolidone crosslinked hydrogels induce wound healing through cell proliferation and migration. Journal of Biomaterials and Tissue Engineering. 2017;7(4):310-318

[13] Yao Q, Li W, Yu S, Ma L, Jin D, Boccaccini AR, et al. Multifunctional chitosan/polyvinyl pyrrolidone/45S5 Bioglass® scaffolds for MC3T3-E1 cell stimulation and drug release. Materials Science and Engineering: C. 2015;**56**: 473-480. DOI: 10.1016/j.msec.2015. 06.046

[14] Bühler V. Polyvinylpyrrolidone Excipients for Pharmaceuticals: Povidone, Crospovidone and Copovidone. Germany: Springer Science & Business Media; 2005. DOI: 10.1017/ CBO9781107415324.004

[15] Rowe RC, Sheskey P, Quinn M. Handbook of Pharmaceutical Excipients. Argentina: Libros Digitales-Pharmaceutical Press; 2009

[16] Bejaoui M, Galai H, Amara ABH, Ben Rhaiem H. Solubility diagram determination of ibuprofen-PVP solid dispersions obtained by milling. Research Journal of Pharmaceutical Biological and Chemical Sciences. 2017;**8**(1):7-17

[17] Chowdary KPR, Srinivas SV. Effect of polyvinylpyrrolidone on complexation and dissolution rate of β- and hydroxypropyl-β-cyclodextrin complexes of celecoxib. Indian Journal of Pharmaceutical Sciences. 2006;**68**(5): 631-634. DOI: 10.4103/0250-474X.29632

[18] Valero M, Pérez-Revuelta BI, Rodríguez, L. J. Effect of PVP K-25 on the formation of the naproxen: β-ciclodextrin complex. International Journal of Pharmaceutics. 2003;**253** (1-2):97-110. DOI: 10.1016/ S0378-5173(02)00664-6

[19] Teodorescu M, Bercea M. Poly (vinylpyrrolidone)–a versatile polymer for biomedical and beyond medical applications. Polymer-Plastics Technology and Engineering. 2015;**54**(9):923-943. DOI: 10.1080/ 03602559.2014.979506

[20] Regulska K, Regulski M, Wzgarda A, Kotowska A, Ignasiak A, Ćwiertnia B, et al. Does polyvinylpyrrolidone improve the chemical stability of cilazapril in solid state? Iranian Journal of Pharmaceutical Research: IJPR. 2019;**18**(2):579. DOI: 10.22037/ ijpr.2019.1100640

[21] Yu DG, Zhang XF, Shen XX, Brandford-White C, Zhu LM. Ultrafine ibuprofen-loaded polyvinylpyrrolidone fiber mats using electrospinning. Polymer International. 2009;**58**(9):1010-1013

[22] Mishra RK, Datt M, Banthia AK. Synthesis and characterization of pectin/ PVP hydrogel membranes for drug delivery system. Aaps Pharmscitech. 2008;**9**(2):395-403

[23] Wlodarski K, Tajber L, Sawicki W. Physicochemical properties of direct compression tablets with spray dried and ball milled solid dispersions of tadalafil in PVP-VA. European Journal of Pharmaceutics and Biopharmaceutics. 2016;**109**:14-23

[24] del Consuelo ID, Falson F, Guy RH, Jacques Y. Ex vivo evaluation of bioadhesive films for buccal delivery of fentanyl. Journal of Controlled Release. 2007;**122**(2):135-140

[25] Rose PA, Praseetha PK, Bhagat M, Alexander P, Abdeen S, Chavali M. Drug embedded PVP coated magnetic nanoparticles for targeted killing of breast cancer cells. Technology in Cancer Research & Treatment. 2013;**12**(5):463-472

[26] Dowding PJ, Atkin R, Vincent B, Bouillot P. Oil core/polymer shell microcapsules by internal phase separation from emulsion droplets.

II: Controlling the release profile of active molecules. Langmuir. 2005;**21**(12): 5278-5284

[27] Prosapio V, De Marco I, Reverchon E. PVP/corticosteroid microspheres produced by supercritical antisolvent coprecipitation. Chemical Engineering Journal. 2016;**292**:264-275

[28] Dong B, Lim LM, Hadinoto K. Enhancing the physical stability and supersaturation generation of amorphous drug-polyelectrolyte nanoparticle complex via incorporation of crystallization inhibitor at the nanoparticle formation step: A case of HPMC versus PVP. European Journal of Pharmaceutical Sciences. 2019;**138**: 105035. DOI: 10.1016/j.ejps.2019.105035

[29] Guduru R, Liang P, Runowicz C, Nair M, Atluri V, Khizroev S. Magneto-electric nanoparticles to enable field-controlled high-specificity drug delivery to eradicate ovarian cancer cells. Scientific Reports. 2013;**3**:1-8. DOI: 10.1038/srep02953

[30] Gaikwad D, Shewale R, Patil V, Mali D, Gaikwad U, Jadhav N. Enhancement in in vitro anti-angiogenesis activity and cytotoxicity in lung cancer cell by pectin-PVP based curcumin particulates. International Journal of Biological Macromolecules. 2017;**104**:656-664. DOI: 10.1016/j.ijbiomac.2017.05.170

[31] Ajji Z, Maarouf M, Khattab A, Ghazal H. Synthesis of pH-responsive hydrogel based on PVP grafted with crotonic acid for controlled drug delivery. Radiation Physics and Chemistry. 2020;**170**:108612

[32] Risbud MV, Hardikar AA, Bhat SV, Bhonde RR. pH-sensitive freeze-dried chitosan–polyvinyl pyrrolidone hydrogels as controlled release system for antibiotic delivery. Journal of Controlled Release. 2000;**68**(1):23-30

[33] Rasekh M, Karavasili C, Soong YL, Bouropoulos N, Morris M, Armitage D, et al. Electrospun PVP–indomethacin constituents for transdermal dressings and drug delivery devices. International Journal of Pharmaceutics. 2014;**473** (1-2):95-104

[34] Dai XY, Nie W, Wang YC, Shen Y, Li Y, Gan SJ. Electrospun emodin polyvinylpyrrolidone blended nanofibrous membrane: A novel medicated biomaterial for drug delivery and accelerated wound healing. Journal of Materials Science: Materials in Medicine. 2012;**23**(11):2709-2716

[35] Okwuosa TC, Stefaniak D, Arafat B, Isreb A, Wan KW, Alhnan MA. A lower temperature FDM 3D printing for the manufacture of patient-specific immediate release tablets. Pharmaceutical Research. 2016;**33**(11): 2704-2712

[36] Kempin W, Domsta V, Grathoff G, Brecht I, Semmling B, Tillmann S, et al. Immediate release 3D-printed tablets produced via fused deposition modeling of a thermo-sensitive drug. Pharmaceutical Research. 2018;**35** (6):1-12

[37] Perioli L, Ambrogi V, Angelici F, Ricci M, Giovagnoli S, Capuccella M, et al. Development of mucoadhesive patches for buccal administration of ibuprofen. Journal of Controlled Release. 2004;**99**(1):73-82

[38] Sadashivaiah R, Dinesh BM, Patil UA, Raghu KS. Design and in vitro evaluation of haloperidol lactate transdermal patches containing ethyl cellulose-povidone as film formers. Asian Journal of Pharmaceutics (AJP). 2014;**2**(1):43-49

[39] Rao PR, Diwan PV. Formulation and in vitro evaluation of polymeric films of diltiazem hydrochloride and indomethacin for transdermal administration. Drug Development and Industrial Pharmacy. 1998;**24**(4): 327-336

[40] Bothiraja C, Shinde MB, Rajalakshmi S, Pawar AP. Evaluation of molecular pharmaceutical and in-vivo properties of spray-dried isolated andrographolide—PVP. Journal of Pharmacy and Pharmacology. 2009;**61**(11):1465-1472

[41] Gupta P, Bansal AK. Spray drying for generation of a ternary amorphous system of celecoxib, PVP, and meglumine. Pharmaceutical Development and Technology. 2005;**10**(2):273-281

[42] Uzun İN, Sipahigil O, Dinçer S. Coprecipitation of cefuroxime axetil–PVP composite microparticles by batch supercritical antisolvent process. The Journal of Supercritical Fluids. 2011;**55**(3):1059-1069

[43] Prosapio V, Reverchon E, De Marco I. Formation of PVP/nimesulide microspheres by supercritical antisolvent coprecipitation. The Journal of Supercritical Fluids. 2016;**118**:19-26

[44] Zhang W, Zhang CN, He Y, Duan BY, Yang GY, Ma WD, et al. Factors affecting the dissolution of indomethacin solid dispersions. Aaps Pharmscitech. 2017;**18**(8):3258-3273

[45] Nielsen LH, Rades T, Müllertz A. Stabilisation of amorphous furosemide increases the oral drug bioavailability in rats. International Journal of Pharmaceutics. 2015;**490**(1-2):334-340

[46] Kim WK, Kim JS, Shin ME, Baek JS, Kim D, Bucciarelli A, et al. Sustained-released formulation of nifedipine solid dispersion with various polymers. Macromolecular Research. 2020;**28**:553-557

[47] Sharma A, Jain CP. Preparation and characterization of solid dispersions of carvedilol with PVP K30. Research in Pharmaceutical Sciences. 2010;**5**(1):49

[48] Karagianni A, Kachrimanis K, Nikolakakis I. Co-amorphous solid dispersions for solubility and absorption improvement of drugs: Composition, preparation, characterization and formulations for oral delivery. Pharmaceutics. 2018;**10**(3):98

[49] Loh ZH, Samanta AK, Heng PWS. Overview of milling techniques for improving the solubility of poorly water-soluble drugs. Asian Journal of Pharmaceutical Sciences. 2015;**10**(4):255-274. DOI: 10.1016/j.ajps.2014.12.006

[50] Bejaoui M, Galai H, Amara ABH, Rhaiem HB. Formation of water soluble and stable amorphous ternary system: Ibuprofen/β-cyclodextrin/PVP. Glass Physics and Chemistry. 2019;**45**(6):580-588. DOI: 10.1134/S1087659619060130

[51] Gupta P, Kakumanu VK, Bansal AK. Stability and solubility of celecoxib-PVP amorphous dispersions: A molecular perspective. Pharmaceutical Research. 2004;**21**(10):1762-1769

[52] Gupta P, Bansal AK. Ternary amorphous composites of celecoxib, poly (vinyl pyrrolidone) and meglumine with enhanced solubility. Die Pharmazie-An International Journal of Pharmaceutical Sciences. 2005;**60**(11):830-836

[53] Szafraniec J, Antosik A, Knapik-Kowalczuk J, Kurek M, Syrek K, Chmiel K, et al. Planetary ball milling

and supercritical fluid technology as a way to enhance dissolution of bicalutamide. International Journal of Pharmaceutics. 2017;**533**(2):470-479. DOI: 10.1016/j.ijpharm.2017.03.078

[54] Sarma P, Kaur H, Medhi B, Bhattacharyya A. Possible prophylactic or preventive role of topical povidone iodine during accidental ocular exposure to 2019-nCoV. Graefe's Archive for Clinical and Experimental Ophthalmology. 2020;**258**:2563-2565

[55] Bejaoui M, Kalfat R, Galai H. The effect of adding PVP to the binary solid dispersion (indomethacin: kaolin) on the formation of physically stable amorphous drug. Journal of Pharmaceutical Innovation. 2021;**16**:1-11

[56] Watanabe T, Wakiyama N, Usui F, Ikeda M, Isobe T, Senna M. Stability of amorphous indomethacin compounded with silica. International Journal of Pharmaceutics. 2001;**226**(1-2):81-91

[57] Aleanizy FS, Alqahtani F, Al Gohary O, El Tahir E, Al Shalabi R. Determination and characterization of metronidazole–kaolin interaction. Saudi Pharmaceutical Journal. 2015;**23**(2): 167-176

[58] Onyekweli AO, Usifoh CO, Okunrobo LO, Zuofa JD. Adsorptive property of kaolin in some drug formulations. Tropical Journal of Pharmaceutical Research. 2003;**2**(1): 155-159

[59] Giri TK, Badwaik H, Alexander A, Tripathi DK. Solubility enhancement of ibuprofen in the presence of hydrophilic polymer and surfactant. International Journal of Applied Biology and Pharmaceutical Technology. 2010;**1**(2):793-800

[60] Mahapatra AK, Murthy PN, Biswal S, Mahapatra AP, Pradhan SP. Dissolution enhancement and physicochemical characterization of valsartan in solid dispersions with β-CD, HP β-CD, and PVP K-30. Dissolution Technologies. 2011;**18**:39-45

[61] Koh PT, Chuah JN, Talekar M, Gorajana A, Garg S. Formulation development and dissolution rate enhancement of efavirenz by solid dispersion systems. Indian Journal of Pharmaceutical Sciences. 2013;**75**(3):291

[62] Bejaoui M, Oueslati H, Galai H. Ternary solid dispersion strategy for solubility enhancement of poorly soluble drugs by co-milling technique. In: Chitin and Chitosan-Physicochemical Properties and Industrial Applications. Rijeka: IntechOpen; 2021

Section 2

Novel Drug Delivery System

Chapter 4

Self-nano Emulsifying Formulations: An Encouraging Approach for Bioavailability Enhancement and Future Perspective

Sunil T. Galatage, Rahul Trivedi, Durgacharan A. Bhagwat, Arehalli S. Manjappa, Swapnil S. Harale, Abhinandan A. Alman, Swapnil S. Chopade, Sujit A. Desai, Shashikant Adsule, Ashish M. Phutane, Samruddhi S. Kadam, Shruti R. Mandekar, Amruta M. Chougale, Krushnabai R. Margale, Rohini M. Patil, Shweta N. Kalebere and Amolkumar A. Kempwade

Abstract

Currently lipid-based formulations are playing a vital and promising role in improving the oral bioavailability of poorly water-soluble drugs. Lipid based formulations mainly consist of a drug dissolved in lipids such as triglycerides, glycerides, oils and surface active agent. Self nanoemulsifying formulations (SNEF) are isotropic mixtures of lipids/oils, surfactants and co-surfactants. On mild agitation followed by dilution in aqueous media, such as GI fluids, SNEF can form fine oil-in-water (o/w) nanoemulsions. Present chapter summarizes different types of lipid formulations with special emphasis on SNEF, availability of dosage forms, different components with natural surfactants from medicinal plants, mechanism of SNEF, recent advancements in oral drug delivery, solid SNEDDS, patents on SNEF and future prospects. SNEF emerging as powerful technique to improve solubility and commercialization of solid SNEF is the future novel drug delivery to improve bioavailability of poorly water soluble drugs.

Keywords: lipid formulation, self nano emulsifying drug delivery system, natural surfactants, ternary phase diagram

1. Introduction

In recent years, promising efforts have been made to use the potentials of lipid drug delivery systems for solubility and bioavailability enhancement potential. Poorly water-solubility and bioavailability are major challenge in front of formulation of scientists in development of new formulation. Lipid-based drug delivery systems (LBDDS) have great potential of versatility and biocompatibility. Lipid-based formulations modified in different routes to adapt a broad range of products as per the requirements of disease and route of administration. The key factor of LBDDS is their safety and efficacy during design and development of medicines [1]. Recently LBDDS gained much importance in reducing variable food effects and enhancement of bioavailability of poorly water-soluble active pharmaceutical ingredient (API). LBDDS offers great advantages like controlled and targeted drug delivery, stability of developed formulation which is capable of carrying both lipophilic and hydrophilic drugs within it [2]. Lipid formulations classified in to liquid lipid-based formulations, emulsions or microemulsion, Self-emulsifying drug delivery systems (SEDDS), solid-in-oil (S/O) suspension, solid lipid-based formulations, lipid as particulate drug carriers, liposome, solid lipid nanoparticles (SLNs), neosome. Present work gives an overview of Self nano-emulsifying formulations, its components, future perspectives and applications in commercialization. SNEF is the most promising approach which overcomes poor water solubility; bioavailability and formulation difficulties poorly water-soluble drugs [3]. SNEF designed to increase solubility and bioavailability of drugs belonging to the BCS Class II-IV. SNEF comprehensively enhance the solubility and bioavailability of poorly water soluble drugs (PWSDs) by micelle formation. In SNEF API introduced as nano-sized oil droplets. Rapid drug release of SNEF in the stomach due to the generation of nanosized oil droplets leads to the quick onset of action in the GI tract. SNEF easily dispersible due to the partitioning of a drug between oil and water which generates a larger interfacial area. SNEF offers ample of advantages such as reproducible plasma drug conc., decrease in variability of rate and extent of absorption [4]. SNEF holds the drug in a solution that allows enough time for drug absorption through GIT [5].

2. Self nano emulsifying formulations (SNEF)

SNEF is an isotropic mixture of surfactants, lipids, and solubilizers having great ability to form fine O/W nano-emulsion by mild agitation. It has droplet size 2–200 nm dispersion in water which improves increase the rate of dissolution and bio-availability of PWSDs [6]. SNEF is the most stable emulsion due to the partitioning of the drug between the oil and aqueous phase gives larger interfacial area. It is technically proven that droplet size of nanoemulsions was not affected by the fed and fasted dissolution conditions. Optimized nanoemulsions reduce bioavailability ratio in fed and fasted state which maintain reproducible plasma profile. Optimized formulation improves oral absorption of PWSDs hence the onset of action is quick. Nanoemulsion improves conc. of the drug in systemic circulation (bioavailability) which leads to a reduction of does and higher does related adverse effects in case of potential anticancer drugs [7].

2.1 Advantages of self nanoemulsifying formulations (SNEF)

1. Nanoemulsion (SNEF) has a much large surface area and free energy.

2. SNEF improve the bioavailability [8].

3. SNEF protects the drug from enzymatic degradation and hydrolysis by dissolving large quantity in lipids and make them suitable carrier for parental transport.

4. SNEF provide large O/W interfacial area and ultra-low interfacial tension

5. SNEF improves low aqueous solubility, low permeability, gastric irritation, enzymatic degradation, and stability.

6. Site specificity and targeted drug delivery can be achieved with SNEF [9].

2.2 Disadvantages of self nanoemulsifying formulations (SNEF)

1. Formulation of SNEF is expensive in recent years due to technological development in a high-pressure homogenizer and ultrasonic equipment of high coast [10].

2. Storage conditions temperature and Ph affects stability [11].

3. Composition of SNEF

3.1 Lipid/oil phase

Choice of specific lipid phase has critical importance in the formulation of optimized SNEF. Maximum capacity of lipid to solubilize selected drug and high drug loading

General class	Examples	Commercial name
Lipids	Soya lipid,Polyoxy- 35 castor oil	Accutane soft gelatin capsule, Cremophor EL
MCTs	Triglycerides of capric acids Triace tin	Miglyol,Labrafac crodamol, Captex, Captex
Medium-chain mono and diglycerides	Capric acids -Mono- and diglycerides	Capmul, Akoline
Mono-glycerides (Long-chain)	GMO-Glyceryl monooleate	Maisine,Peceol, GMO-Capmul
Polyethylene Glycol (Fatty acids esters)	Polyethylene Glycol monolaurate/dilaurate Polyethylene Glycol dicaprylate/caprate	Capryol, capmul, Sefsol Lauroglycol, capmule, lauroglycol Migylol, captex
Esters fatty acid	Isopropyl myristate	Crodamol EO
Fatty acids	Caprylic acid	Crossential
Vitamins	Vitamin E D-alpha TocopherylPoly ethylene Glycol1000 Succinate (Vit.E-TPGS)	Tocofersolan

Table 1.
Commonly used oils in SNEF.

General class	Examples	Commercial name
Polysorbates	Sorbitan monolaurate	Tween 80, crillet 4
Sorbitan esters	Sorbitan monolaurate	Span 20,68,80, Crill 1,3,4
Copolymers	Poloxamer 188 and 407	Pluronic F-68 and F 127
Castor oil	Castor oil	Cremphor, Etocas
Polyglycolyzed glycerides	Linoleoyl macrogol glycerides Oleoyl macrogol glycerides Caprylocapryol macrogol glycerides Polyglyceryl oleate Lauroyl macrogol glycerides Stearoyl macrogyl glycerides	Labrafil, Labrasol, Plurol oleique, Gelucire, Gelucire
Phospholipids	Soybean / sunflower lecithin	ALCOLEC®

Table 2.
Commonly used surfactants in SNEF [14].

capacity are the major criteria for selections of lipid for the development of nanoemulsion. Oil phase has a great ability to increase drug loading capacity for transport of drug in systemic circulation by an increase in absorption of PWSDs [12]. Omega oil is essential fatty acids that the human body needs for metabolic functioning. Human body needs Essential Fatty acids (EFAs) to remove toxic harmful waste products, cell membrane repair and to get optimum nutrition. Main objective of EFAs to generate prostaglandins which controls functions such as blood pressure, heart rate, regulating inflammation, blood clotting etc. Omega oil also helps in treatment of breast, colon and prostate cancer [13]. Some are mentioned in **Table 1**.

3.2 Surfactants

For design and development of optimized SNEF large no. of compounds have properties of surfactants but few orally acceptable such as nonionic surfactants having low HLB. A large number of surfactant is associated with toxicity. Hence the safety is a major concern while a selection of Surfactant molecule (**Table 2**) [12].

4. Solubilizers

Solubilizers are incorporated in nanoemulsions to increase drug loading capacity to modulate droplet size and self emulsification time of optimized formulation (**Table 3**) [15].

General class	Examples
Alcohols (Short-chain)	C2H5OH
Alkame (Diols and Triols)	PEG
Polyethylene glycols	PEG 400
Glycol ethers	Diethylene glycol monoethyl ether(transcutol)

Table 3.
Commonly used solubilisers in SNEF [16].

5. Mechanism of SNEF

In nanoemulsions, entropy change favors dispersion as compared to the energy required to increase the surface area of dispersion. SNEF mainly involves surface free energy which is used by nanoemulsion to produce new surface area in oil and water system can be represented in following equation

$$\Delta G = \sum N \pi r^2 \sigma \quad (1)$$

Where ΔG is the surface free energy associated, N is the number of droplets of radius r and ó represents the interfacial energy [17]. Emulsifying agent stabilizes the emulsion when two phases immiscible concerning time to decrease interfacial area. In nanoemulsions, coalescence is avoided due to droplets of monolayer which reduce interfacial energy required for the formulation of nanoemulsion. Free energy required for formulations is low, positive or negative [18].

6. SNEF and recent advancements in oral drug delivery

SNEF is a recent advancement in lipid-based nanoemulsions and it is a promising strategy to solubilize drug molecule in the lipid phase which is biocompatible. SNEF play dual function it protects entrapped drug molecule against degradation in GI fluids also absorption of the drug in lymphatic transport increased. It mainly focused on the impact on the size and surface nature of nanocarriers on targeted uptake by entrecote [19, 20]. **Figure 1** shows an overview of encapsulated SNEF developed for oral administration. SNEF expressed as to potential nanoemulsion which is thermodynamically and kinetically more stable hence it has great ability to enhance oral bioavailability of PWSDs [21]. In 1995 for first-time saquinavir was introduced in the market in salt form having only 4% bioavailability in a hard gelatin capsule. After 02 years bioavailability increased 03 folds in human by formulating in SNEF with medium-chain mono- and diglycerides [22, 23].

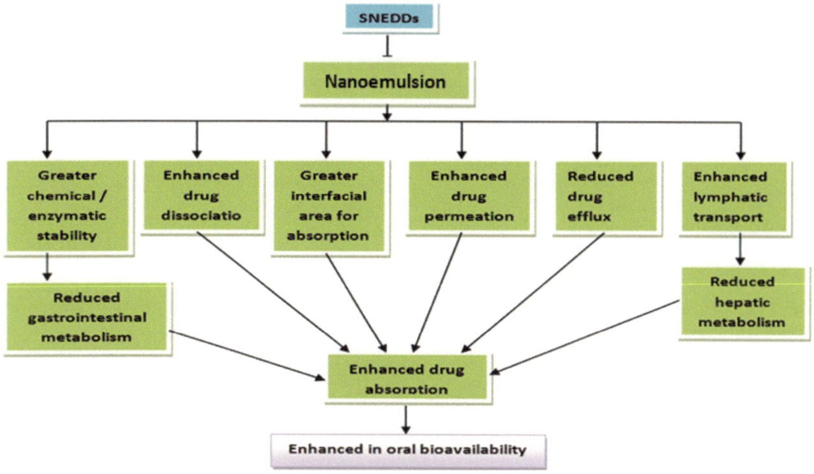

Figure 1.
Enhancement of oral bioavailability through SNEF.

7. Phase diagram of lipid formulations

The phase diagram in SNEF is constructed to choose a right potential candidate of oil, surfactant, and co-surfactant which is selected by varying concentration of surfactant, oil, and solubilizers depending on physiochemical properties of API such as surface activity and polarity. Orange colored area of self good self emulsification are established by diluting the mixture of oil and surfactant sequentially phase studies are performed by an increase in the amount of water (**Figure 2**). Once equilibrium is achieved types of phases recognized by using an optical microscope or cross-polarized viewer [24, 25].

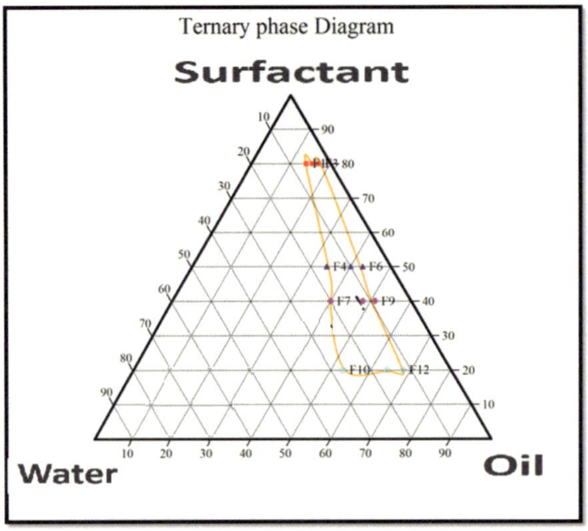

Figure 2.
Schematic ternary phase diagram of SNDDS system.

8. Methods of preparation of nanoemulsion

(Figure 3)

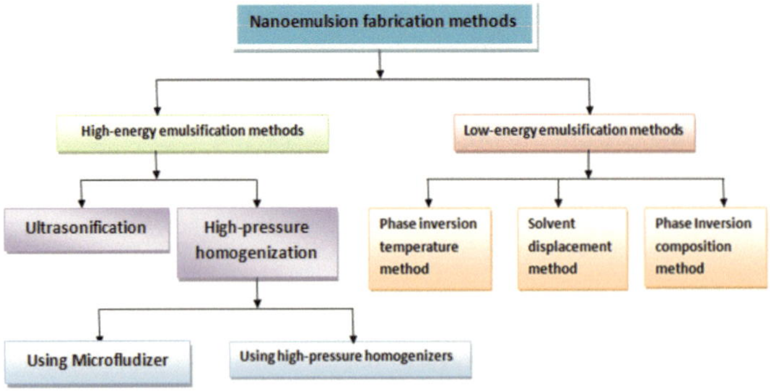

Figure 3.
Methods of Preparation of Nanoemulsions.

9. *In vitro-in vivo* correlation (*IVIVC*) for self nanoemulsion

New drug synthesis and design, optimization of new drug and its formulations are very costly and time consuming processes and *IVIVC* play prime importance in it. Optimization demands *in vivo* bioequivalence data in human to ascertain similarity of the new formulation. Due to this load importance of performing bioequivalence studies significantly increase hence coast of formulation and optimization process increases. To solve this problem it is necessary to perform in vitro tests that can interpret bioavailability data. *IVIVC* concept was established in scientific research studies which give a prediction of in-vitro parameter with in vivo activity [26, 27]. The *IVIVC* predominantly used in the product development to decrease the human trials during the formulation development and to support biowaivers. *IVIVC* acts as vital tool for correlating *in vitro* and *in vivo* data. Core balance of *IVIVC* study in development and optimization of new formulation with minimum human trials [28]. *IVIVC* is a mathematical model which predicts the relation between rate and extent of drug release and plasma drug concentration. For drugs that are administered orally, dissolution and intestinal permeation are considered as the rate-limiting steps for the absorption. Bioavailability is calculated by controlling dissolution profile, therefore, if an excellent correlation exists between *in vitro* dissolution test and a bioavailability parameter, then controlling the dissolution profile will permit the evaluation of bioavailability [29]. The *in vitro* drug release studies of the formulations can be performed using dissolution, disintegration tests on t other hand *in vivo* pharmacokinetic study performed on animal models. Apart from this, there is a limited number of *IVIVC* studies conducted using lipid formulations. To get strong *IVIVC* relationship a large no. of nanoemulsions of PWSDs administered orally. Clinical data of more human volunteers along with in detail evaluation of in-*vitro* and *in vivo* solubility of poorly water soluble drugs entrapped in lipid vehicles [30].

10. Solid SNEF

As Nanoemulsions facing problems related to stability, handling, formulation and development scientist decided to overcome these hurdles related to stability and converted nanoemulsions into solid-state and concept of solid SNEF coined. Solid dosage forms are most convenient and stable for handling and they are dry solid powder overcomes hurdles of stability. Adsorption on a solid carrier is the best technique involved to convert liquid nanoemulsion to solid SNEF apart from other techniques available such as spray drying and freeze-drying. The choice right process for the formulation of solid SNEF Mainly depends on the properties of API, such as solubility, stability, and compatibility with other ingredients and nature of the oil phase of the formulation. Adsorption on the surface of adsorbent act as a binder and it is coast effective, accurate, optimizable, uncomplicated and large scale manufacturing is possible with ease. Adsorption on solid carrier adsorbs heat and moisture sensitive drugs can be formulated into SNEF also it has an advantage over other methods. Commonly used adsorbents in SNEF are Neusilin-US2, Fujicalin, Aerosil etc. [31].

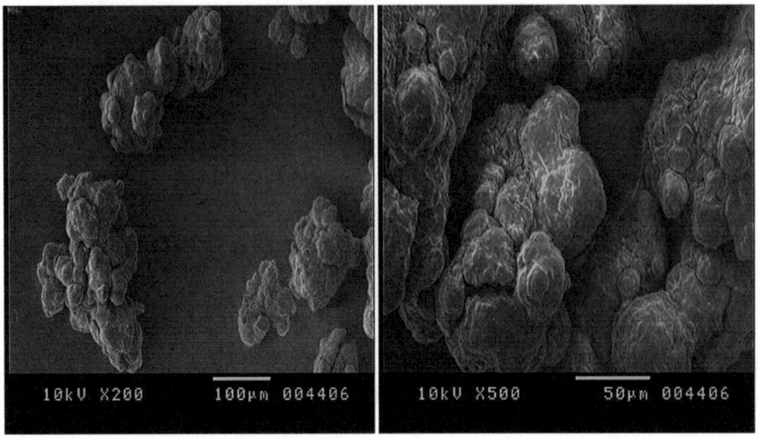

Figure 4.
SEM of SNEF adsorbed on neusilin-US2 adsorbant.

10.1 Ideal characteristics of an adsorbent

1. Adsorb viscous, sticky and oily nanoemulsions

2. Compatible, safe, freely flow able, high bulk density,

3. Should not alter dissolution profile once converted to solid form.

Researchers developed and characterized solid nanoemulsion granules (SNGs) of ezetimibe and ezetimibe-simvastatin in combination by using aerosol 200 as adsorbent. Results of X-ray diffraction shows improvement in the solubility of drugs in SNGs. Scanning electron microscopy indicates no precipitation of drug on the surface carrier. Drastic enhancement in dissolution profile of the drug in SNGs when compared to pure drug. Plasma level data in rats show a significant decrease in total cholesterol level compared to pure drug (**Figure 4**).

10.2 Evaluation of SNEF

- Thermodynamic stability studies
- Robustness to dilution
- Assessment of Efficiency of self-emulsification
- % Transmittance
- Viscosity
- Dye solubilization test
- Cloud point measurement

Drug	Therapeutic use	Components	In vitro/in vivo observation
B-lactamase	A model protein	Hydrogenated lecithin, Cremophor EL, Transcutol, lauroglycol FCC	2–3-fold BA increment compared with the solution
Biphenyl dimethyl dicarboxylate	Hepa to protection	Tween 80, transcutol, Miglyol 812	1.7–6-fold improvement in BA
Cyclosporine A	Immunosuppressant	Cremophor EL, Capmul, MCM C8, Orange oil	Improvement in dissolution rate
Anethole trithione	Chemopreventive	Tween 80, PG, cremophor RH 40 MCT	Improved stability and in vitro dissolution profile

Table 4.
Potential of SNEF in oral drug delivery.

10.3 SNEF: Potential explored

Self nanoemulsions have a unique capability to improve therapeutic effectiveness oral bioavailability of PWSDs which is proved by various in-vitro-in-vivo methodologies. Pharmacodynamic efficacy of drugs improved by formulating PWSDs in nanoemulsions. The solubility of PWSDs in different lipids, surfactants, and solubilizers along with their compatibility is key factors while the successful formulation of SNEF [32]. The key investigations that describe the potential of SNEF in oral drug delivery are listed in **Tables 4** and 5.

11. Applications of SNEF

11.1 Bioavailability and solubility improvement

Drug of Class-II drug (Low solubility/high permeability) and formulated in SNEF, then it increases the solubility. Ketoprofen is a non-steroidal anti-inflammatory drug (NSAIDs), mainly it is used for sustained release formulation. In chronic therapy ketoprofen cause gastric irritation due to its low solubility its release from sustained formulations is incomplete. As ketoprofen developed in nanoemulsion complete drug release form sustained formulation of ketoprofen achieved successfully. Ketoprofen developed in SNEF producing oil in water O/W emulsion, droplets of nanoemulsion make drug available for absorption in dissolved form in GIT.Many different approaches available to achieve sustained release which causes decrease in irritation and increase in bioavailability such as matrix pallets, nanocrystals, micro particles, floating oral system apart from these SNEF found upper hand over these [33].

11.2 Protection against biodegradation

SNEF enhance absorption due to larger surface area, reduction in surface area; reduce degradation of PWSDs having both low oral bioavailability and poor water solubility due to degradation of drug by enzymatic degradation and acidic Ph in stomach.

Patent No.	Agency	Year	API	Lipid/Oil	Surfactant
US2013/0303495A1	United State Patent	2013	Testosterone	Castor Oil	Cremophor RH40, Imwotor 742
US8728518B2	United State Patent	2014	Butylpthalide	Castor Oil, Almond Oil, Oleic acid	Cremophor EL,Labrafac CM10,Labrasol M1944,Mabrafil M2125CS
W02014/205226A1	World Intellectual Property Organization	2014	Progesterone, Fenofibrate	Castor Oil, Polysorbate-20,40,60	Propylene Glycol, Monocaprylate Glyceryl Mono caprylate
W02014/009434A1	World Intellectual Property Organization	2014	Abiraterone	Corn Oil, Olive Oil, Sunflower Oil	Labrafac, Captex, PEG
W02015/142307A1	World Intellectual Property Organization	2015	Rosuvastatin	Oleic Acid	Labrasol, Labrafil M1944, Transcutol.
W02016/141098A1	World Intellectual Property Organization	2016	Ophthalmic Drugs	Castor Oil, Olive Oil, Sunflower Oil	Labrafac, Captex, PEG
WO2017/017649A1	World Intellectual Property Organization	2017	Astaxanthin	Akoline CM C	Labrasol, Tween 80
US9918965B2	United State Patent	2018	Diindolylmethane	Peppermint Oil	Gelucire, Capryol, Polysorbate 80
W02018/011808A1	World Intellectual Property Organization	2018	Cannabinoids	Castor Oil	Polysorbate 80, PEG 1000

Table 5.
Patents of SNEF.

11.3 Solid SNEF

Self emulsifying formulations adsorbed on solid carrier and converted in to free flowing power which may filled in to capsule or compressed in to tablet with suitable excipients. To overcome stability related problems of nanoemulsions these are adsorbed on adsorbents to convert them in solid dosage forms tablet or capsule [34].

11.4 SNEF for TCM

Silybin protects liver cells from damage of drinking, smoking and liver-damaging drugs. Due to low solubility of silybin in water it has very low bioavailability when given orally. Hence when silybin formulated in SNEF with ethyl linoleate as lipid, Tween and dimethyl isosorbide as surfactant and co-surfactant respectively bioavailability of silybin increased 04 folds.

12. Future perspectives

In recent years modernization in SNEF research drastically enhance solubility and oral bioavailability of poorly water soluble moieties. The conversion of liquid to a solid SNEF drastically reduces the drug degradation rate. Therefore, it has vital importance to study novel tools and techniques to enhance bioavailability drugs. With help of sophisticated equipment's and modern techniques liquid SNEF converted to a solid form including tablets and pellets. Modern adsorbents like neusilin-US2 should be used for converting liquid SNEF into a solid powder without change in physio-chemical properties of drug along with increase in volume and density [35].

13. Conclusions

Approximately 40% newly synthesized drug moieties are associated with poor water solubility, low bioavailability, high intra- and inter-subject variability, and a lack of dose proportionality. SNEF is now becoming a promising approach to enhance solubility, dissolution and hence bioavailability of poorly water-soluble drugs. An additional advantage of SNEF over simple oily solutions is that they provide a large interfacial area for the partitioning of the drug between oil and water. Incorporation of a liquid SNEF into a solid dosage form may combine the advantages of SNEF with those of a solid dosage form and overcome the disadvantages of liquid formulations. Conclusively, SNEF would be a promising approach for poorly water soluble drugs to improve its therapeutic interventions.

Acknowledgements

The authors are thankful to Department of Pharmaceutics Sant Gajanan Maharaj College of Pharmacy Mahagaon and Trustees of Sant Gajanan Maharaj College of Pharmacy Mahagaon for providing required guidance and support for completion of this work.

Conflict of interest

The authors declare no conflict of interest.

Notes/thanks/other declarations

Special thanks to **Shivtej S. Galatage** for his countionous support throughout the work.

List of abbreviations

SNEF	Self nano-emulsifying Formulations
O/W	Oil-in-water

LBDDS	Lipid-based drug delivery systems
API	Active pharmaceutical ingredient
PWSDs	Poorly water soluble drugs
SLNs	Solid Lipid Nanoparticles
EFAs	Essential Fatty acids
IVIVC	In vitro in vivo correlation
SNGs	Solid nanoemulsion granules
NSAIDs	Non-steroidal anti-inflammatory drug

Author details

Sunil T. Galatage[1,2*], Rahul Trivedi[2], Durgacharan A. Bhagwat[3], Arehalli S. Manjappa[4], Swapnil S. Harale[1], Abhinandan A. Alman[1], Swapnil S. Chopade[4], Sujit A. Desai[5], Shashikant Adsule[1], Ashish M. Phutane[1], Samruddhi S. Kadam[1], Shruti R. Mandekar[1], Amruta M. Chougale[1], Krushnabai R. Margale[1], Rohini M. Patil[1,6], Shweta N. Kalebere[6] and Amolkumar A. Kempwade[7]

1 Sant Gajanan Maharaj College of Pharmacy, Mahagaon, Maharashtra, India

2 B.R. Nahata College of Pharmacy, Department of Pharmacy, Mandsaur University, Mandsaur, Madhya Pradesh, India

3 Bharati Vidyapeeth College of Pharmacy, Kolhapur, Maharashtra, India

4 Tatyasaheb Kore College of Pharmacy, Warana-nagar, Maharashtra, India

5 Annasaheb Dange College of D Pharmacy, Ashta, Maharashtra, India

6 Genesis Institute of Pharmacy, Radhanagari, Maharashtra, India

7 KLE's College of Pharmacy, Nipani, Karnataka, India

*Address all correspondence to: gsunil201288@gmail.com

References

[1] Shrestha H, Bala R, Arora S. Lipid-based drug delivery systems: A review. Journal of Pharmaceutics. 2014;**1**:1-10

[2] Shivhare UD, Chopkar PT, Bhusari KP. Effect of formulation variables on pharmacotechnical properties of carvedilol self-emulsifying drug delivery. Research Journal of Pharmaceutical Dosage forms and Technology. 2009;**1**(3):275-279

[3] Mohshin K. Lipid-based nano delivery for oral administration of poorly water-soluble drugs (PWSDs) design, optimization, and in-vitro assessment. Advanced Technology for Delivering Therapeutics. 2017;**3**:31-51

[4] Souto EB, Muller RH. Informa healthcare. Nanoparticulate Drug Delivery Systems. 2007;**166**:45-56

[5] Gonnade YR, Niranjane K, Ambatkar A. Lipid: An emerging platform for lipid-based drug delivery system: A review. World Journal of Pharmacy and Pharmaceutical sciences. 2014;**3**(4):572-589

[6] Raghuveer P, Vanithakamal J, Madhuri D. Design development and evaluation of self nanoemulsifying drug delivery system of simvastatin. Research Journal of Pharmacy and Technology. 2018;**11**(3):1185-1192

[7] Savale SK. Self nano emulsifying drug delivery system (SNEDDS): A review. International Journal of Research in Pharmaceutical and Nano Sciences. 2015;**4**(6):385-397

[8] Chenmala K, Sureshkumar R, Upadhyay D. Formulation development and In vitro characterization of solid self nano emulsifying drug delivery system for curcumin to target colon adenocarcinoma. Research Journal of Pharmacy and Technology. 2019;**12**(7):3338-3346

[9] Ghadge D, Yadav A, Gharge V. Design and development of solid self microemulsifying durg delivery of Gefitinib. Asian Journal of Pharmacy and Technology. 2018;**4**(8):193-199

[10] Dixit RP, Nagarsenker MS. Formulation and *in vivo* evaluation of self-nano emulsifying granules for oral delivery of a combination of ezetimibe and simvastatin. Drug Development and Industrial Pharmacy. 2008;**34**:1285-1296

[11] Dange V, Shid S, Magdum CS. A review: Dry emulsion. Asian Journal of Pharmaceutical Research. 2015;**5**(4):208-210

[12] Strickley RG. Solubilizing excipients in oral and injectable formulations. Pharmaceutical Research. 2004;**21**:201-230

[13] Gowda KP, Gurav G. Role of omega fatty acids in human body. Asian Journal of Researach in Chemistry. 2009;**2**(2):93-99

[14] Patel PA, Chaulang GM, Hdrdikar SR. Self emulsifying drug delivery system: A review. Research Journal of Pharmacy and Technology. 2008;**1**(4):313-323

[15] Date AA, Nagarsenker MS. Parenteral microemulsions: An overview. International Journal of Pharmaceutics. 2008;**355**:19-30

[16] Makadia HA, Bhatt AT, Paun JS. Self-nano emulsifying drug delivery system (SNEDDS): Future aspects. Asian Journal of Pharmaceutical Research. 2013;**3**(1):20-26

[17] Sonawale P, Patil A, Bhutkar M. Solubility enhancement of lipophilic drugs-solid self micro-emulsifying drug delivery system. Asian Journal of Pharmacy and Technology. 2016;**6**(3):155-158

[18] Pouton C, Porter C. Formulation of lipid-based delivery systems for oral administration: Materials, methods, and strategies. Advanced Drug Delivery Reviews. 2008;**60**(6):625-637

[19] Shahba AA, Mohsin K, Alanazi FK. Novel self-nano emulsifying drug delivery system (SNEDDS) for oral delivery of cinnarizine: Design, optimization, and *in Vitro* assessment. AAPS PharmSciTech. 2012;**13**(3):967-977

[20] Mohsin K. Development of self-nano emulsifying drug delivery systems for the enhancement of solubility and oral bioavailability of fenofibrate, a poorly water-soluble drug. International Journal of Nanomedicine. 2016;**11**:2829-2838

[21] Cerpnjak K. Lipid-based systems as a promising approach for enhancing the bioavailability of poorly water-soluble drugs. Acta Pharmaceutica. 2013;**63**(4):427-445

[22] Perry CM, Noble S. Saquinavir soft-gel capsule formulation. A review of its use in patients with HIV infection. Drugs. 1998;**55**(3):461-486

[23] Hoffmann LR. Fortovase (saquinavir) soft gelatin capsules. Product Information. 2003;**20**:8-14

[24] Ninjawade BK. Functions of lipids for enhancement of oral bioavailability for poorly water-soluble drugs. Scientia Pharmaceutica. 2011;**79**:705-727

[25] Uppoor VR. Regulatory perspectives on *in vitro* (dissolution)/*in vivo* (bioavailability) correlations. Journal of Controlled Release. 2001;**72**(1-3):127-132

[26] Ghosh P, Milewski M, Paudel K. *In vitro/in vivo* correlations in transdermal product development. Therapeutic Delivery. 2015;**6**(9):1117-1124

[27] Anand O. Dissolution testing for generic drugs: An FDA perspective. The AAPS Journal. 2011;**13**(3):328-335

[28] Hwang SS, Bayne W, Theeuwes F. *In vivo* evaluation of controlled release products. Journal of Pharmaceutical Sciences. 1993;**82**(11):1145-1150

[29] Abd-Elbary A, Tadros MI, Alaa-Eldin AA. Development and *in vitro/in vivo* evaluation of etodolac controlled porosity osmotic pump tablets. AAPS PharmSciTech. 2011;**12**(2):485-495

[30] Mohsin K, Long MA, Pouton CW. Design of lipid based formulations for oral administration of poorly water-soluble drugs: Precipitation of drug after the dispersion of formulations in aqueous solution. Journal of Pharmaceutical Sciences. 2009;**98**(10):3582-3595

[31] Dixit RP, Nagarsenker MS. Selfnanoemulsifying granules of ezetimibe: design, optimization, and evaluation. European Journal of Pharmaceutical Sciences. 2008;**35**:183-192

[32] Date AA, Desai N. Self nano emulsifying drug delivery system: Formulation insights, applications, and advances. Nanomedicine. 2010;**5**(10):1595-1616

[33] Bhagwat DA, D'Souza JI. Formulation and evaluation of solid self micro emulsifying drug delivery system using aerosil 200 as a solid carrier. International Current Pharmaceutical Journal. 2012;**1**:414-419

[34] Daga AS, Ingole BD, Kulkarni SS. Self emulsifying drug delivery system:

Hitherto and Novel approach. Research Journal of Pharmacy and Technology. 2012;**5**(6):736-745

[35] Galatage ST. Self-emulsifying drug delivery system: A novel tool to enhance the solubility of poorly water-soluble drugs. International Journal of Pharmacy Practice and Drug Research. 2019;**9**(2):25-32

Chapter 5

Novel Topical Drug Delivery Systems in Ophthalmic Applications

Ankita Rajput, Palvi Sharma, Ritika Sharma and Shubham Thakur

Abstract

The eye is the utmost attention-grabbing organ owed to its drug disposition characteristics. Generally, topical application (90% are eye drops) is the method of choice because of its patient compliance and safety. Transcorneal penetration is the major route for ophthalmic drug absorption. However, corneal absorption has been observed to be slower process as compared to elimination. Therefore, conventional dosage forms are associated with rapid precorneal drug loss. Thus, to improve ocular drug bioavailability, there is a substantial effort directed toward the development of novel topical drug delivery systems for ophthalmic administration. These novel delivery systems (Contact lenses, *In situ* gels, Microemulsions, Niosomes, Liposomes, Implants, Microspheres, and Micelles) provide the controlled release behaviour for treating the chronic ailments, and help patients and doctors to curtail the dosing frequency and invasive method of treatment. Hence, the current chapter discusses the progress of novel topical ocular drug delivery systems in the pharmaceutical industry.

Keywords: ophthalmic, topical delivery, contact lenses, *In situ* gels, microemulsions, niosomes, liposomes, implants, microspheres, micelles

1. Introduction

Eye is the utmost attention-grabbing organ owed by its drug disposition characteristics. Drug delivery to the eye is hampered by the physiological barricades such as blinking & wash out by tears, nasolacrimal drainage, nonproductive losses, and impermeability of the cornea [1, 2]. Although its easy to administer the drug to eyes but there are various barriers to drug delivery, viz. tear mechanisms, membranes, and blood–aqueous and blood–retinal barriers [3]. The three main routes for administering ophthalmic medication are topical, systemic, and intraocular; each has its own set of benefits and drawbacks.

Topical application (90 percent of which are eye drops) is the preferred method due to patient compliance and safety. The most common route for ophthalmic drug absorption is through transcorneal penetration. Corneal absorption, on the other hand, is a much slower process than elimination. Despite the benefits of ocular formulations (ease of formulation, storage limitations, and drug instillation), they have several drawbacks, including limited drug accumulation for lipophilic agents, precorneal losses, and the cornea's barrier [4]. As a result, traditional ocular dosage forms have been linked to rapid precorneal drug loss. Effective systemic delivery, can be achieved if high drug concentration circulates in the blood plasma. Furthermore, sustained release of oral drugs may be appropriate for glaucoma patients, allowing for continuous and effective treatment; butin this method the entire body is exposed to the drug, so, side effects can be observed [5]. Moreover, intravitreal drug delivery is an invasive procedure that carries some risk, such as retinal haemorrhage or detachment, especially if the technique is repeated multiple times for treating chronic disorders.

Traditional eye drops are convenient and easy method, but they are ineffective, and only a small portion of the dose is delivered to the target area; the majority is lost owing toclearance mechanisms. As a result, there are significant strategies aimed at developing novel topical drug delivery systems for ophthalmic administration in order to improve ocular drug bioavailability. Solubility enhancers are primarily used to increase the drug concentrations within the formulation; medication in the dosage form enhances the bioavailability. This strategy may allow for the application of a smaller droplet, and loss due to the reflex tearing and blinking can be prevented to larger extent [5]. Second, the formulation can be designed to withstand clearance; these dosage forms are retained for longer periods of time, giving them more time to remain accumulated within the ocular tissue. Finally, drug penetration enhancers can be added to the formulation to help the drug get through the cornea [6]. All of these approaches are novel drug delivery technologies that allow drugs to reach the posterior chamber. These delivery systems viz. contact lenses, *in situ* gels, microemulsions, niosomes, liposomes, implants, microspheres, and micelles provide controlled release for the treatment of chronic eye disorders, reducing dose frequency and invasive treatment.

Following that, the chapter looks at how novel topical ocular drug delivery systems are progressing in the pharmaceutical industry. Future research is likely to lead to the discovery of polymers that outperform those currently in use, such as smart drug delivery systems that release their payload in response to a specific stimulus. Furthermore, a reassess of recent advances in ophthalmic drug delivery necessitates and aids drug delivery scientists in modulating their thought processes and developing novel and safe drug delivery techniques. Its goal is to sumup the existing traditional ocular delivery formulations and their advancements, as well as current developments. In addition, recent advancements in novel ocular drug delivery strategies, such as contact lenses, *in situ* gels, microemulsions, niosomes, liposomes, implants, microspheres, and micelles have been thoroughly discussed.

2. Dosage forms for topical ophthalmic drug delivery systems

2.1 Conventional therapy

2.1.1 Topical

Topical ocular administration is one of the most often used traditional ways for treating problems of the eye's anterior structures, such as the pre-ocular, cornea, anterior, and posterior chambers. It has four major advantages over other delivery methods: (i) effects of drugs are localised, and very less drug enters the systemic circulation; (ii) it enhances the drug absorption into the eye, which is otherwise difficult to accomplish with systemic administration of drugs; (iii) it bypasses hepatic first-pass metabolism; and (iv) it is a relatively convenient, and painless way of administration. Despite its numerous advantages, topical drug delivery have limited bioavailability due to the numerous biological processes that exist to protect the eye and, as a result, limit the entry of ocular medications [7].

2.1.2 Eye ointments

Ointments are typically made from a combination of semisolid and solid hydrocarbons (paraffin), having a melting or softening point near body temperature and donot cause irritation to the eyes. Simple bases, in which the ointment forms a single continuous phase, or compounded bases, in which a two-phased system (e.g., an emulsion) is used, are the two types of ointments. The medicinal substance is either introduced as a solution or as a finely micronised powder to the base. Ointments break down into little droplets after being injected into the eye, and they stay in the cul-de-sac for a long time as a drug depot. As a result, ointments are useful for increasing bioavailability and sustaining release of drug. Ointments, despite being safe and well tolerated by the eye, have low patient compliance due to blurred vision and occasional discomfort [8].

2.1.3 Gel

Gel formation is a uniquecase of viscosity enhancement using viscosity enhancers, which leads to longer pre-corneal residence period. It provides benefits such as lower systemic exposure. Despite its extremely high viscosity, gel only improves bioavailability to a limited extent, and dose frequency can be reduced to once a day at most. The excessive viscosity, on the other hand, causes hazy vision and matted eyelashes, which significantly reduces patient acceptance. Polymers including polyacrylamide, poloxamer, carbomer, poly methylvinylethermaleic anhydride, and hydroxypropyl ethylcellulose are commonly used in aqueous gels. Controlled drug delivery systems are made up of swellable water insoluble polymers, known as hydrogels, or polymers with unusual swelling properties in aqueous medium. Most ofently swellings are observed when drugs are released through these systems via transport of solvent into the polymer matrix. Diffusion of the solute through the inflated polymer leads to erosion/dissolution in the final stage. In humans, a poly (acrylic acid) hydrogel has been shown to considerably increase tropicamide ocular bioavailability when compared to a paraffin ointment and viscous solution [9]. Pilopine HS® gel, introduced by Alcon in 1986, and more recently Merck's Timoptic-XE®.

2.1.4 Intravitreal injection

Many debilitating and sight-threatening disorders are caused by posterior segment diseases, and the only method to cure them is through invasive treatments such as "intravitreal injection" In most cases, this is still true, although advances have resulted in a broad variety of viable implantable drug-delivery systems for diseases of posterior segment, and the several possibilities will now be explored. Injection into the vitreous humour of eye is the most popular method of placing drugs in the posterior chamber; this gives a high concentration of drug where it is needed while minimising systemic effects. Xu *et al.,* found that the diffusion of polystyrene nanoparticles of different sizes and surface chemistries in fresh bovine vitreous humour and found that depending on the nanoparticle's intended features, they were able to achieve adequate drug transport within the posterior chamber [10]. However, many disorders, such as cataracts, retinal detachment, haemorrhage, endophthalmitis, and ocular hypertension, necessitate frequent treatment, which can lead to intraocular complications.

This approach includes injecting a medication solution into the vitreous through the pars plana using a 30G needle, which improves drug absorption over systemically and topically administered drugs. It results in drug distribution to the eye's target areas. Drug delivery to the posterior segment of the eye is much safer as compared to systemic mode of drug administration. Intravitreal injection, as opposed to other methods, gives larger medication concentrations in vitreous and retina. Following intravitreal delivery, a drug's molecular weight determines how quickly it is eliminated [11]. Despite the fact that intravitreal delivery provides high drug concentrations in the retina, it is linked to a number of short-term problems, including retinal detachment, endophthalmitis, and intravitreal haemorrhages [12]. Patients must also be closely watched during intravitreal injections. It has disadvantages like first-order kinetics (this rapid rise may cause toxicity, and drug efficacy can diminish as the drug concentration falls below the targeted range), injections have a short half-life (a few hours), and they must be given repeatedly, and side effects like pain from repeated injections, discomfort, increased IOP, intraocular bleeding, increased infection risks, and the risk of retinal detachment.

2.1.5 Emulsions

A vast range of lipophilic medicines have been employed to treat eye problems in recent years. Oil-in-water emulsions have improved significantly bioavailability to ophthalmic region.. Yamaguchi *et al.,* combined a 0.05 percent w/v difluprednate (DFBA) ocular lipid emulsion with 5.0 percent castor oil and 4.0 percent polysorbate 80 to make a 0.05 percent w/v DFBA ophthalmic lipid emulsion [13]. At 1 hour after instillation, the lipid emulsion had a 5.7-fold greater concentration of DFB, an active metabolite of DFBA, in the aqueous humour than the DFBA ophthalmic suspension. The first time this product was sold in the United States was in 2008. Shen et al. created an ocular emulsion of flurbiprofenaxetil (FBA), a well-known NSAID, and discovered that the mean retention time (MRT) of flurbiprofen in aqueous humour increased as the oil content increased. Flurbiprofen's area under the curve (AUC0–10 h) was 6.7 times higher in the FBA emulsion group than in the FBA oil solution group. A promising NSAID ophthalmic emulsion with minimal irritancy and increased anti-inflammatory action was found in the nanoparticle with a raised FBA concentration of 0.1 percent [14].

Cationic emulsion changes have been reported to improve spreading capabilities, decrease contact angle, and increase ocular surface residence time. Oleyamine, stearylamine, chitosan, arginine octadecylamine, and 1,2-dioleoyl-3-trimethylammonium-propane are examples of cationic materials (DOTAP). The tear fluid drug levels in the CE were 3.6 and 3.8 times greater than those in the non-coated emulsion (NE) after topical administration of indomethacin-chitosan-coated emulsion (CE) at 0.5 and 0.75 hours, respectively. CE's residence time is 1.5 times longer than NE's [15]. Klang *et al.,* studied indomethacin corneal penetration in anionicsubmicron emulsions, cationic emulsions, and commercially available ocular solutions [16]. Cationic emulsions have four times the spreading coefficients of anionic emulsions. Other emulsions had substantially lower drug levels in aqueous humour and sclera-retina than this new therapy.

2.2 Novel therapies

2.2.1 Contact lenses

Contact lenses are polymeric devices with hydrophilic or hydrophobic charactersitics that are designed toplace directly onto the cornea to correct refractive errors of eye. In comparison to its anhydrous state, hydrogel contact lenses are practical materials for use as ocular medication delivery systems because they can ingest a considerable volume of aqueous solution. If the contact lens hydrating solution has enough pharmaceutically active material, it will be able to diffuse from the polymer matrix into the tear film bathing the eye and interact with the ocular tissue. However, there is still a requirement to keep the medicine in the devices long enough to ensure proper release of drugs.

Wichterle and Lim proposed the notion of employing hydrogel contact lenses as drug-delivery devices in their 1965 patent, which suggested including medication following lens hydration to provide extended drug availability throughout usage [17]. The type of contact lens dictates how it is worn; daily, weekly, and monthly disposable versions are available [17]. The absorption of a drug-loaded solution during pre-wear soaking was used in early efforts to contact lens-assisted drug delivery. Drug distribution through standard contact lenses is inconsistent, with a brief initial "burst release" and then a quick fall. Drug-loaded coating or the insertion of a sandwich layer of drug-loaded polymer, the inclusion of drug-loaded nanoparticles, and cyclodextrin grafting are some of the other techniques. Molecular imprinting technology is a method of modifying polymer formulations to increase their affinity for drug molecules, hence enhancing drug loading potential and extending delivery time [18–20]. Hiratani et al., 2006 used this strategy to construct a system that used methacrylic acid, N, N-diethylacrylamide, and the medication timolol to generate sustained timolol release in vitro for over 48 hours. Alvarez-Lorenzo et al., used the same approach to make norfloxacin-loaded poly (hydroxyethyl methacrylate) (pHEMA) contact lenses, reporting a 300-fold increase in reservoir capacity over pHEMA lenses without molecular imprinting technology [21]. HEMA, mono-methacrylated-cyclodextrin, and trimethylolpropane trimethacrylate were used by Xu et al. [22] to make hydrogel films and contact lenses. Puerarin was used as a model medication by soaking the gel in a drug solution to hydrate it [22]. Loading and release rates were found to be dependent on -cyclodextrin content in in vitro tests. In vivo tests on rabbits revealed that the gels provided better medication release and performance than commercial puerarin eye drops. The researchers believe the material is suitable for drug delivery from reusable daily wear contact lenses because the devices have outstanding mechanical qualities.

2.2.2 Niosomes

Niosomes are nonionic structural vesicles with two layers that can encapsulate both lipophilic and hydrophilic substances. Niosomes boost ocular bioavailability by reducing systemic drainage and increasing residence duration. In nature, they are nonbiodegradable and nonbiocompatible. Niosomal formulation was developed as a new way to distribute cyclopentolate. The medication was released regardless of pH, leading in a considerable increase in ocular bioavailability. A niosomal formulation of coated (chitosan or carbopol) timolol maleate had a significant influence on decreasing IOP in rabbits compared to timolol solution [23].

2.2.3 Microemulsion

Microemulsions are stable water-oil dispersions aided by the use of a surfactant and co-surfactant combination to lower interfacial tension. The drug's ocular bioavailability is improved, and the frequency of administration is reduced, thanks to microemulsion. Higher thermodynamic stability, tiny droplet size (100 nm), and a clean appearance are common characteristics of these systems [24]. An oil-in-water system containing pilocarpine, lecithin, propylene glycol, PEG 200 as a surfactant/co surfactant, and isopropyl myristate as the oil phase did not irritate the rabbit animal model. Such formulations frequently enable continuous medication release, reducing drug delivery frequency. Its stability is affected by the potential toxicity of greater surfactant/co-surfactant concentrations, surfactant/co-surfactant selection, and aqueous/organic phase.

2.2.4 Liposomes

Liposomes are tiny vesicles made up of one or more lipid bilayers separated by water or an aqueous buffer. Liposomes have the ability to make close contact with the corneal and conjunctival surfaces, improving the chances of ocular medication absorption. This capability is especially useful for drugs that are poorly absorbed, have a low partition coefficient, poor solubility, or have a molecular weight of medium to high. The surface charge of liposomes has been discovered to play a role in their behaviour as an ocular medication delivery system. In comparison to neutral or negatively charged liposomes, positively charged liposomes appear to be preferentially trapped at the corneal surface which has negative charged. It has the properties of being droppable, biocompatible, and biodegradable. It decreased the drug's toxicity. It allows for long-term release and site-specific delivery. Liposomes are difficult to make in a sterile environment. It has drawbacks such as a low drug load and poor water stability. Schaeffer *et al.,* found that liposome uptake by the cornea is greatest for positively charged liposomes and least for neutral liposomes when working with indole and penicillin G. This finding suggests that electrostatic adsorption is the initial interaction between the corneal surface and liposomes [25].

2.2.5 Implants

The intraocular implant's purpose is to provide sustained activity with regulated medication release from the implant's polymeric substance. The implants must constantly be administered intraocular, which necessitates minimal surgery. They are usually implanted intravitreal, at the pars plana of the eye (abruptly anterior to the retina and posterior to the lens) [26, 27]. Despite the fact that this is an invasive procedure, the implants have the advantages of (1) delivering consistent therapeutic doses of medication straight to the site of action by avoiding the blood-ocular barrier, (2) avoiding the negative effects linked to repeated intravitreal and systemic injections, and (3) requiring a smaller amount of drug during treatment. Ocular implants are divided into two categories: non-biodegradable and biodegradable.

Non-biodegradable implants can enable more precise medication release control and longer release times than biodegradable polymers, but they require surgical implant removal, which comes with its own set of dangers.

The delivery rate of implants could be controlled by changing the polymer composition. Solid, semisolid, or particulate-based delivery systems can be used to deliver implants. There are typically three phases to the drug release from polylactic acid, polyglycolic acid, and polylactic-co-glycolic acid: an initial burst, a middle diffusive phase, and a final burst of the drug. It's a better option to repeated injections because it extends the drug's half-life and may help to reduce peak plasma levels; it may also enhance patient acceptance and amenability. It has drawbacks, such as side effects: the insertion of these devices is invasive, and there are ocular complications that come with it (retinal detachment and intravitreal haemorrhage for intravitreal implant). Once the device has been depleted of the drug, it must be harvested through surgery (risk of ocular complications). The drug release profile of the biodegradable implants has an uncontrollable final burst [27].

2.2.6 *In situ-forming gel*

When the droppable gels are instilled, they become liquid and then transition to a viscoelastic gel in the ocular cul-de-sac, providing a response to environmental changes. It raises the level of patient acceptance. It extends the drug's time in the eye and improves its ocular bioavailability. pH, temperature, and ionic strength are all variables that can affect and trigger the phase transition of droppable gels. Gelling is caused by a variety of factors, including a change in pH, which causes CAP latex cross-linked polyacrylic acid and its derivatives, carbomers and polycarbophil, a change in temperature, which causes poloxamers, methyl cellulose, and Smart HydrogelTM, and a change in ionic strength, which causes Gelrite and alginate [28–31].

2.2.7 *Microspheres*

It has been described how erodible, non-erodible, and lipid microspheres can be used for ophthalmic delivery. The drug is uniformly dispersed (monolithic system) in the polymer matrix. Due to this, the drug may or may not be present in the liquid carrier medium in which the drug-loaded microparticles are suspended. Pilocarpine-loaded gelatin and albumin microspheres were released and pharmacokinetic data were presented by Leucatta *et al.,* in 1989. Hardened proteinaceous microspheres with a diameter of about 30 pm produced biphasic release of pilocarpine over a period of two to five days. Drug recovery was reported to be around 20% in gelatin and 28% in albumin microspheres. The colloidal system outperformed the aqueous control in terms of significant pharmacokinetic parameters.

Furthermore, the lipid microspheres significantly increased intraocular steroid penetration when compared to non-detectable or no penetration with suspension. The release of proteins of various sizes, including lysosome, trypsin, heparinize, ovalbumin, albumin, and immunoglobin, from poly(anhydrides) microspheres (50–125 pm) and poly(anhydrides) copolymers has been reported [32]. Fatty acid dimer and sebacic acid were copolymerized in various ratios with various molecular weights to create microspheres. The particle size, cross linking density, and drug loading all influence the in vitro release of drugs from microspheres. For a week, these microspheres generated release rates that were nearly constant or zero. The liquid medium in which the microparticles are suspended should have a pH and osmolarity that are acceptable to the eye, and the dosage form should be soothing and non-irritating to the user. Additionally, neither the polymer nor its degradants should be harmful to the eyes [33].

2.2.8 Micelles

Amphiphilic surfactants or diblock polymers are used to make micelles. Recently, the efficacy of a polyion complex micelle system incorporating a dendritic phtalocyanine photosensitizer in photodynamic therapy of choroidal neovascularization was tested in rats. Absorption at 650 nm was observed in the micellar system, which is advantageous for the treating deep lesions. The formulation may be able to selectively accumulate in choroidal neovascularized lesions and extend bloodstream retention, but these possibilities will need to be further investigated [34–36].

3. Advantages of novel over conventional topical ophthalmic drug delivery systems

The delivery of ophthalmic drugs is one of the most difficult tasks confronting pharmaceutical researchers. Their target is to achieve and maintain a therapeutic level at the action site for a long time. To keep medication levels at the target site for an extended period of time, novel drug delivery methods should be created. In terms of distinct delivery methods or tools to be used before, during, or after administration, novel drug delivery systems are fresh on the market and variations on earlier ones. Existing remedies are becoming ineffective as a result of the development of new technology. By decreasing drug exposure to non-target cells and increasing the amount and durability of a drug around target cells, new drug delivery methods improve a drug's therapeutic effects while minimising its harmful consequences [37]. One of the most difficult delivery methods for pharmaceutical researchers is ophthalmic medication delivery [38]. Traditional delivery methods like suspensions, solutions, emulsions, intravitreal injections, and ointments have poor ocular bioavailability, or less than 1%, as a result of various factors including fast yield, low absorption, short residence time in the cul-de-sac, and relatively impermeable drugs [39]. Within 5 minutes of administration, up to 80% of the administered dose may be lost due to tears and nasolachrymal drainage. **Figure 1** illustrates the difference between conventional and novel drug delivery systems.

The use of viscosity enhancers, ophthalmic solutions in which the drug dissolves slowly, or ophthalmic inserts can all be used to extend the duration of therapy [37]. Because it prolongs drug release and allows for greater contact with the front of the eye, ophthalmic drug administration is optimal [38]. Novel ocular drug administration aims to prolong medicine retention duration in the eye or facilitate transcorneal drug penetration to boost drug bioavailability [40]. From eye drops to ophthalmic iontophoresis, in situ gels, dendrimers, ocular inserts mucoadhesive polymers, penetration enhancers, mucoadhesive polymers, hydrogels, and targeted drug delivery systems, topical ocular medication delivery has been enhanced [41]. Most frequently available ophthalmic preparations are eye drops and ointments. Nonetheless, due to tear flow and lachrymal nasal drainage, these preparations are rapidly drained away from the ocular cavity when instilled into the cul-de-sac. Because only a small amount is available for therapeutic effect, frequent dosing is required. Over the past three

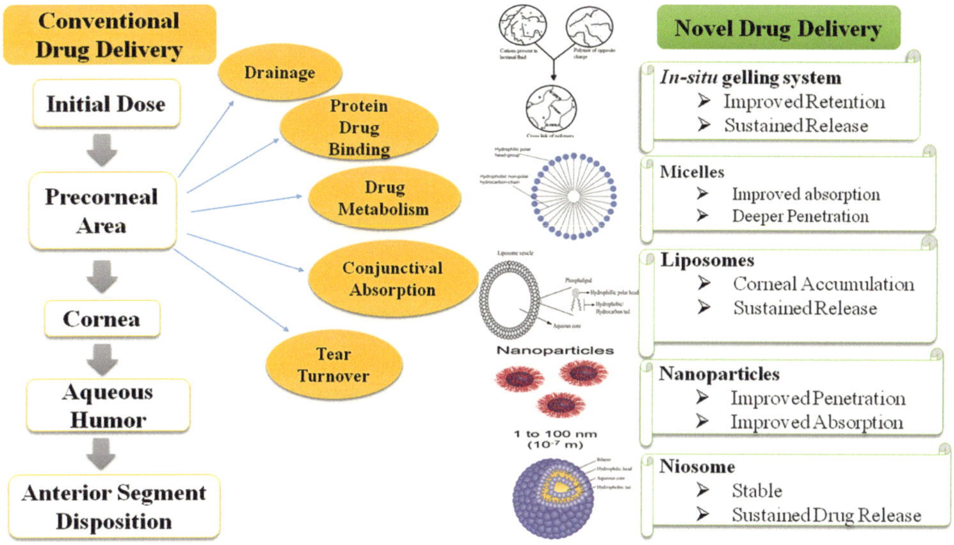

Figure 1.
Advantages of novel drug delivery systems over conventional systems in ophthalmic applications.

decades, newer pharmaceutical ophthalmic formulations have been created to address these problems. These formulations include in situ gel, nanoparticle, liposome, nanosuspension, microemulsion, iontophoresis, and ocular inserts [42].

4. Harmonious additives and their role in novel topical ophthalmic drug delivery systems

4.1 Poloxamer

A thermoresponsive polymer called poloxamer begins as a liquid between 4 and 5°C and in a concentration range of 20 to 30% wt/wt before changing to a gel when the temperature of the medium increases. When used alone, higher concentrations of Poloxamer are necessary in a formulation; nevertheless, such amounts have been shown to irritate the eyes. In order to reduce the overall amount of Poloxamer utilised, enhance the gelling and mechanical properties of Poloxamer, and lower the risk of eye irritation, Poloxamer was combined with other polymers such methyl cellulose, chitosan, and others [43]. Poloxamers, also known as Pluronics, are tri-block copolymers made up of poly (ethylene oxide), poly (propylene oxide), and poly (ethylene oxide) (PEO-PPO-PEO). Kolliphor P188 (also known as Poloxamer 188 or Pluronic F-68) has roughly 27 PPO groups on one side and 80 PEO groups on the other. Kolliphor P188 has a molecular weight of about 8400 g mol1, which is higher than that of normal emulsifying surfactants [44]. Below 50°C, it exists as single molecules (unimers) and at higher temperatures polymolecular micelles starts to form. These can be used in a wide range of occular drug delivery applications due to the variety of microemulsion types created [45].

4.2 PLA: PCL: PEG: PCL: PLA copolymers

Endophthalmitis, impaired vision, increased cataract formation, intraocular pressure, and an elevated vulnerability of retinal detachment are all side effects of numerous intravitreal corticosteroid injections, which are induced by maintaining sustained levels of corticosteroids in the case of maculae edoema. Copolymers can be used to lessen these undesirable effects. Recently, there has been a lot of interest in amphiphilic block copolymers based on biodegradable polyesters like poly-caprolactone (PCL) and polyethylene glycol (PEG) [46]. PEG is a typical component in block copolymers as the hydrophilic section. PEG is a promising medication delivery material because of its high water solubility and minimal cytotoxicity [47]. PCL is a thermoplastic polyester that is biocompatible, biodegradable, and nontoxic. Its segments may come together to form a hydrophobic core that serves as a storage space for drugs that are insoluble in water [46].

Perret and his colleagues were the first to develop a series of PEG and PCL block copolymers [48]. Since then, numerous experiments on PCL and PEG-based di and tri-block copolymers have been done. Gong and coworkers formulated honokiol-loaded PEGPCL-PEG micelles using a direct dissolution method assisted by ultrasonication [49]. Lue *et al* created a thermosensitive PEG–PCL–PEG hydrogel and investigated its ability for diclofenac sodium ocular medication delivery (DIC) [50]. Peng and colleagues looked into the use of PEG-PCL-PEG hydroge in rabbits as an intracameral implant to prevent scarring after surgery. They discovered that the prolonged release of bevacizumab from the hydrogel reduced neovascularization and scar formation [51]. Furthermore, due to the high crystallinity of PCL blocks, tri-block copolymers based on PCL appear to have limits in terms of biodegradability and drug release [49].

4.3 PLGA

The poly lactic-co-glycolic acid (PLGA) copolymer comprising poly lactic acid (PLA) and poly glycolic acid (PGA), which is employed in medical applications such surgical sutures, bone plates and screws, tissue engineering scaffolds, and drug carrier systems, has been successfully created [52]. The mechanical characteristics of poly lactic-co-glycolic acid (PLGA), a biocompatible, biodegradable, and tunable polymer, can be changed by varying the molecular weight and PLA/PGA ratio. When utilised for medicine delivery, PLGA is hydrolyzed in vivo to produce biodegradable metabolite monomers such lactic acid and glycolic acid, which have very low systemic toxicity [53].

The use of PLGA-based-NPs for ocular drug administration has several advantages, including protection of encapsulated pharmaceuticals against fast inactivation, delayed drug release owing to polymer breakdown (e.g. Ciprofloxacin-loaded PLGA), and surface modification to target specific regions or cells. For example Flurbiprofen was loaded in PLGA nanoparticles with Poloxamer 188, diclofenac-loaded PLGA nanoparticles and flurbiprofen-loaded nanoparticles are used against ophthalmic anti-inflammatorydisorders and enhanced permeability of inflamed area [54]. Additionally, hydrophilic or hydrophobic medications as well as macromolecules, proteins, peptides, and nucleic acids can be efficiently encapsulated in PLGA nanoparticles [55].

4.4 Vitamin E TPGS

Chemically, vitamin E TPGS is polyethylene glycol-esterified vitamin E succinate (PEG-1000). The chemical composition of TPGS is classified as a surfactant with no charges on its surface; the hydrophilic head section is separated from the lipophilic tail portion by an alkyl group. The well-known adjuvant TPGS has been employed in a variety of medicinal compositions. The word "TPGS" refers to an oil-soluble vitamin also known as tocopherols and tocotrienols. Tocopherol, a naturally occurring vitamin, is the one with the highest potency [56]. As an antioxidant, vitamin E TPGS works to reduce oxidative stress, which has been associated to a number of eye conditions, including glaucoma, age-related macular degeneration, uveitis, and cataracts. Age-related disorders are most frequently brought on by oxidative stress, despite the fact that the exact aetiology is uncertain. As a result, TPGS may be a great alternative to conventional drugs in treating these conditions, acting as a neuroprotectant in age-related diseases [57].

In order to increase drug translocation in the cornea, TPGS can be utilised in conjunction with transdermal medication delivery because low water solubility of medications restricts their pharmacological effects for eye illnesses and limits their penetration. Cholkar *et al.* used TPGS and octoxynol-40 to make dexamethasone-loaded micelles. When compared to TPGS (0.025 wt percent) and Oc-40, the combined polymers had a reduced CMC (0.012 wt %) (0.107 wt %). The cytotoxicity of the formulations on rabbit primary corneal epithelial cells demonstrated their safety [58]. Rapamycin-loaded micelles were also created using TPGS and Oc-40, and in vitro tests on human retinal pigment epithelium and rabbit primary corneal epithelial cells demonstrated that they were well tolerated and barely harmful. Additionally, the micelles demonstrated clinical viability, exhibiting modest drug partition into vitreous fluid but very high drug concentrations at the retina-choroid target region [59].

In recent years, TPGS has been studied for ocular disorders along with several drugs such as cyclosporine (a micellar system was produced using Poloxamer and vitamin E TPGS to enhance drug concentration during delivery);curcumin (formulated with Pluronic P123 (P123) and vitamin E TPGS to increase permeation across cornea); rapamycin (formulated using vitamin E TPGS and octoxynol-40 to enhance its water solubility); acyclovir (formulated with vitamin E TPGS and octoxynol-4 to slow the release of drug and site specific absorption); riboflavin (to improve riboflavin penetration across the cornea even without removing the epithelium); dexamethasone (formulated with polylactide-co-glycolide (PLGA) and vitamin E TPGS to decrease the limitations of the posterior segment drug delivery); dorzolamide (to overcome the problem of frequent instillation) and timolol (to enhance intraocular pressure reduction capability of contact lens even at lower dose) [57].

4.5 Cyclodextrin

Cyclodextrins are oligosaccharides with a hydrophilic outer surface and a lipophilic interior chamber that can form water-soluble complexes [60]. When applied topically, cyclodextrin nanoparticles promote mucoadhesion, I increase the concentration of dissolved medicine in the eye drop and subsequently in tear fluid, (ii) and (iii) allow drug molecules transit through the unstirred water layer immediately close to the eye surface [10, 61, 62]. Tanito et al. [61] examined the impact of nanoparticle-cyclodextrin dexamethasone eye drops on diabetic macular oedema and discovered a notable decrease in retinal thickness and an improvement in visual acuity, with outcomes comparable to those attained with intravitreal therapy [63].

Cyclodextrins are cyclic oligosaccharides that form complexes with lipophilic medicines to boost their solubility. Cyclodextrin interactions with biological membranes have also been discovered to play a part in their efficacy in increasing solubility. The number of Cyclodextrins used for solubility improvement is quite important.

Large quantities can reduce bioavailability by holding medicine in tears; ideally, 15% or less should be supplied [64, 65]. Some of the eyedrops that contain Cyclodextrins that are registered in Europe are chloramphenicol (Clorocil®: Edol), diclofenac (Voltaren Ophthalmic®: Novartis), and indomethacin (Indocid®: Merck Sharp & Dohme-Chibret).

Topical medication administration to the anterior and posterior segments based on cyclodextrin has been claimed to have the ability to overcome physio-anatomical limitations, as well as the inadequacies and side effects associated with ocular drug delivery [66]. The use of cyclodextrin inclusion complex to boost the drug molecule's water solubility has been widely questioned, leading in a rise in the number of formulations on the market that use cyclodextrin as an excipient. Cyclodextrins are cyclic oligosaccharides formed naturally when starch is digested by bacteria. Compared to linear dextrin, the structure of –1,4-glyosidic connections of -D glucopyranose units is cyclic, making it more resistant to non-enzymatic degradation. When compared to fungizon, cyclodextrin improved issolution and penetration when combined with dexamethasone or ilomastat, and its combination with amphotericin raised antifungal activity by 35 times [67].

4.6 Carbopol

Carbopol, carbomer, and acrylic acid polymers are polymers of acrylic acid with allyl sucrose or allyl ethers of pentaerythritol that are synthesised at high molecular weight [68]. Each can be used as a bioadhesive component, controlled release agent, emulsifying agent, emulsion stabiliser, rheology modifier, or stabilising agent in ophthalmic formulations [69]. The -blockers timolol, betaxolol, carteolol, and metipranolol were combined with carbopol to create a formulation that was demonstrated to be particularly successful in lowering intraocular pressure [70]. Each one may be utilised in ophthalmic formulations as a bioadhesive component, controlled release agent, emulsifying agent, emulsion stabiliser, rheology modifier, or stabilising agent.

Carbopol has also been utilised in Gel-Larmes-Thea formulations to treat dry eye syndrome [71]. When the pH exceeds its pKa, a sol-to-gel transition occurs in aqueous solution, and the reaction to shear strain is Newtonian time-dependent. The nonlinear synthetic nonlinear polymers that make up the carbopol resins (910, 934, 940, 941, and 962) mostly consist of acrylic acid and are cross-linked with a polyalkenyl polyether. Johnson et al. demonstrated the effectiveness of carbopol in extending corneal residence time in rabbits by injecting pilocarpine nitrate into their eyes [72]. The bioadhesive properties of carbopol are another advantage, as they can increase viscosity and, consequently, residence time. They can also form potent non-covalent bonds with the mucin that covers biological membranes and remain there for a similar amount of time.

4.7 Polysorbate 80

Tween 80 and Polysorbate 80 are both non-ionic polyethoxylated (PEO) sorbitan monooleates [45]. It is composed of a copolymer of sorbitol oleate ester and its anhydrides, in which 20 mol of PEG are added for every mole of sorbitol and its anhydrides [73]. A sorbitan ring is connected to four hydrophilic PEO head groups for a total of 20. In the hydrophobic area, an ester couples an oleyl, unsaturated tail to one PEO group [74]. The kink in Polysorbate 80's hydrophobic tail allows for flexibility, resulting in an ideal curvature and packing characteristic for microemulsion production [75]. In rabbits, the oil in water emultion formulation of Difluprednate combined with Polysorbate 80 aids in the stabilisation of a greater dose in the aqueous humour than the suspension formulation [13].

4.8 PEG-40 hydrogenated Castor oil

Cremophors are polyethoxylated castor oils produced by reacting varying concentrations of hydrogenated castor oil with ethylene oxide. To create PEG-40 hydrogenated castor oil, 40 mol of ethylene oxide are combined with 1 mol of hydrogenated castor oil. Glycerol polyethylene ricinoleate is the hydrophobic portion of such surfactants, while polyethylene glycols and glycerol ethoxylates are the hydrophilic portion [76]. PEG-40 hydrogenated castor oil is predominantly made up of hydrophobic elements, the most prominent of which being glycerol polyethylene glycol 12-hydroxystearate [76]. The HLB value is still high (14–16), and its water solubility has increased, as a result of the many hydrophilic polyethylene oxide (PEO) groups. As a result, PEG-40 hydrogenated castor oil can function as an oil solubilizer as well as an o/w microemulsion emulsifier [45]. Cyclosporine is combined with hydrogenated castor oil to provide a topical ophthalmic medication with improved solubility [77].

5. Action plan and future prospective

As indicated by the literature from the pharmaceutical engineering, medical, and academic domains, an action plan to sustain future breakthroughs and clinical success is necessary to channel the increased interest in this topic. To continue these discussions and see the successful application of more drug delivery systems in ophthalmology, we propose: (i) increased collaboration at academic institutions between basic and applied scientific teams, where many novel drug delivery systems are discovered; (ii) collaboration between pharmaceutical corporations and researchers in basic and applied sciences to speed up technology transfer and enable the creation and sale of innovative prions; (iii) standardised procedures for collecting ocular tissue samples for pharmacokinetic comparisons. Samples of posterior ocular tissues like the choroid, retinal pigment epithelium, neuroretina (macula and peripheral retina), and sclera should be obtained consistently to improve data comparison; (iv) To help sponsors choose the best route to regulatory approval of innovative ocular drug delivery systems, there should be clear guidelines, including early and regular communication with regulatory bodies; (v) gatherings and organisations that foster conversation between fundamental, applied, and clinical researchers in order to support upcoming joint efforts in the creation of medical devices and drugs as well as in ophthalmology translational research; (vi) Rewards for participating persons and organisations; (vii) Journals that support and welcome translational research papers in subjects including the outcomes of preclinical testing, the creation of analytical techniques, plans for the advancement of investigational medications, and critical evaluation of trials that fall short of their objectives.

6. Conclusion

Drug distribution to ocular tissues has been a significant problem for ocular scientists for many years. The use of drug solutions as topical drops with conventional formulations had some drawbacks, prompting the development of new carrier systems for ocular delivery. Huge efforts are being made in ocular research to develop novel drug delivery strategies that are both safe and patient-friendly. Researchers are currently working hard to improve the in vivo performance of conventional formulations. On the other hand, ocular scientists are intrigued by the development of nanotechnology, innovative methods, gadgets, and their applications in drug delivery. Using invasive, non-invasive, or minimally invasive drug administration techniques, drug molecules are encapsulated in particulate or vesicular carrier systems or devices.

Contact lenses, in situ gels, microemulsions, niosomes, liposomes, implants, microspheres, and micelles are just a few of the nanotechnology-based carrier systems being developed and studied. A few of these are mass-produced commercially and used in clinical settings. The body of the patient gains from novel medication delivery methods by lowering drug-induced toxicity and visual loss. Additionally, these carriers or devices lengthen drug release, increase targeted moieties' specificity, and help reduce dose frequency. However, after non-invasive medication administration, a carrier system that can reach targeted ocular tissue, including the tissues in the rear of the eye, is still required to be developed. A topical drop formulation that maintains a high precorneal residence time, prevents non-specific drug tissue buildup, and delivers therapeutic drug levels into targeted ocular tissue is anticipated at the current rate of ocular research and development (both anterior and posterior). Invasive drug delivery techniques like intravitreal and periocular injections may one day be replaced by this delivery technology.

Conflict of interest

Author(s) confirms that, there are no conflicts of interest.

Author details

Ankita Rajput[1], Palvi Sharma[1], Ritika Sharma[2] and Shubham Thakur[3]*

1 Department of Botanical and Environmental Sciences, Guru Nanak Dev University, Amritsar, Punjab, India

2 Sri Sai College of Pharmacy, Pathankot, Punjab, India

3 Department of Pharmaceutical Sciences, Guru Nanak Dev University, Amritsar, Punjab, India

*Address all correspondence to: shubhamdthakur@gmail.com
and shubhamdpharma.rsh@gndu.ac.in

References

[1] Tseng CL, Chen KH, Su WY, Lee YH, Wu CC, Lin FH. Cationic gelatin nanoparticles for drug delivery to the ocular surface: In vitro and in vivo evaluation. Journal of Nanomaterials. 2013;**2013**:1-7

[2] Gupta H, Aqil M, Khar RK, Ali A, Bhatnagar A, Mittal G. Sparfloxacin-loaded PLGA nanoparticles for sustained ocular drug delivery. Nanomedicine nanotechnology, biol med. Nanomedicine. 2010;**6**:324-333

[3] Yasukawa T, Tabata Y, Kimura H, Ogura Y. Recent advances in intraocular drug delivery systems. Recent Patents on Drug Delivery & Formulation. 2011;**5**:1-10

[4] Abdulrazik M, Behar-Cohen F, Benita S. Drug Delivery Systems for Enhanced Ocular Absorption. Enhancement in drug delivery. 2007;**24**:1-10

[5] Washington N, Washington C, Wilson CG. Physiological Pharmaceutics: Barriers to Drug Absorption. New York: Taylor & Francis; 2001

[6] Nagarwal RC, Kant S, Singh PN, Maiti P, Pandit JK. Polymeric nanoparticulate system: A potential approach for ocular drug delivery. Journal of Controlled Release. 2009;**136**:2-13

[7] Davies NM. Biopharmaceutical considerations in topical ocular drug delivery. Clinical and Experimental Pharmacology & Physiology. John Wiley & Sons, Ltd. 2000;**27**:558-562

[8] Sasaki H, Yamamura K, Mukai T, Nishida K, Nakamura J, Nakashima M, et al. Enhancement of ocular drug penetration. Critical Reviews in Therapeutic Drug Carrier Systems. Begel House Inc. 1999;**15**:85-146

[9] Giannaccini B, Alderigi C. Semisolid ophthalmic vehicles. Bollettino Chimico Farmaceutico. 1989;**128**:257-266

[10] Xu Q, Boylan NJ, Suk JS, Wang YY, Nance EA, Yang JC, et al. Nanoparticle diffusion in, and microrheology of, the bovine vitreous ex vivo. Journal of Controlled Release. 2013;**167**:76-84

[11] Marmor MF, Negi A, Maurice DM. Kinetics of macromolecules injected into the subretinal space. Experimental Eye Research. 1985;**40**:687-696

[12] Ausayakhun S, Yuvaves P, Ngamtiphakorn S, Prasitsilp J. Treatment of cytomegalovirus retinitis in AIDS patients with intravitreal ganciclovir. Journal of the Medical Association of Thailand. 2005;**88**:15-20

[13] Yamaguchi M, Yasueda SI, Isowaki A, Yamamoto M, Kimura M, Inada K, et al. Formulation of an ophthalmic lipid emulsion containing an anti-inflammatory steroidal drug, difluprednate. International Journal of Pharmaceutics. 2005;**301**:121-128

[14] Shen J, Gan L, Zhu C, Zhang X, Dong Y, Jiang M, et al. Novel NSAIDs ophthalmic formulation: Flurbiprofen axetil emulsion with low irritancy and improved anti-inflammation effect. International Journal of Pharmaceutics. 2011;**412**:115-122

[15] Yamaguchi M, Ueda K, Isowaki A, Ohtori A, Takeuchi H, Ohguro N, et al. Mucoadhesive properties of chitosan-coated ophthalmic lipid emulsion containing indomethacin in tear fluid. Biological & Pharmaceutical Bulletin. 2009;**32**:1266-1271

[16] Klang S, Abdulrazik M, Benita S. Influence of emulsion droplet surface charge on indomethacin ocular tissue distribution. Pharmaceutical Development and Technology. 2000;**5**:521-532

[17] Wichterle O, Lim D. Cross-linked hydrophilic polymers and articles made therefrom. United States Patent Official. 1965;**3220960**:3-6

[18] Byrne ME, Park K, Peppas NA. Molecular imprinting within hydrogels. Advanced Drug Delivery Reviews. Elsevier. 2002;**54**:149-161

[19] Salian VD, Vaughan AD, Byrne ME. The role of living/controlled radical polymerization in the formation of improved imprinted polymers. Journal of Molecular Recognition. John Wiley & Sons, Ltd. 2012;**25**:361-369

[20] White CJ, Byrne ME. Molecularly imprinted therapeutic contact lenses. Expert Opinion on Drug Delivery. Informa Healthcare. 2010;**7**:765-780

[21] Alvarez-Lorenzo C, Yañez F, Barreiro-Iglesias R, Concheiro A. Imprinted soft contact lenses as norfloxacin delivery systems. Journal of Controlled Release. 2006;**113**:236-244

[22] Xu J, Li X, Sun F. Cyclodextrin-containing hydrogels for contact lenses as a platform for drug incorporation and release. Acta Biomaterialia. 2010;**6**:486-493

[23] Sahoo SK, Dilnawaz F, Krishnakumar S. Nanotechnology in ocular drug delivery. Drug Discovery Today. 2008;**13**:144-151

[24] Ansari MJ, Kohli K, Dixit N. Microemulsions as potential drug delivery systems: A review. PDA Journal of Pharmaceutical Science and Technology. 2008;**62**:66-80

[25] Schaeffer HE, Krohn DL. Liposomes in topical drug delivery. Investigative ophthalmology & visual science. 1982;**22**:220-227

[26] Bourges JL, Bloquel C, Thomas A, Froussart F, Bochot A, Azan F, et al. Intraocular implants for extended drug delivery: Therapeutic applications. Advanced Drug Delivery Reviews. 2006;**58**:1182-1202

[27] Yasukawa T, Ogura Y, Sakurai E, Tabata Y, Kimura H. Intraocular sustained drug delivery using implantable polymeric devices. Advanced Drug Delivery Reviews. 2005;**57**:2033-2046

[28] Schmidt PC. Encyclopedia of pharmaceutical technology. Vol. 1; Eds. J. Swarbrick and J. C. Boylan, M. Dekker, Inc. New York 1988, 494 p. hardcov. Price: See review text. Pharmazie in Unserer Zeit. John Wiley & Sons, Ltd. 1990;**19**:130

[29] Steinfeld A, Lux A, Maier S, Süverkrüp R, Diestelhorst M. Bioavailability of fluorescein from a new drug delivery system in human eyes. The British Journal of Ophthalmology. 2004;**88**:48-53

[30] Hume LR, Lee HK, Benedetti L, Sanzgiri YD, Topp EM, Stella VJ. Ocular sustained delivery of prednisolone using hyaluronic acid benzyl ester films. International Journal of Pharmaceutics. 1994;**111**:295-298

[31] Cohen S, Lobel E, Trevgoda A, Peled Y. A novel in situ-forming ophthalmic drug delivery system from alginates undergoing gelation in the eye. Journal of Controlled Release. 1997;**44**:201-208

[32] Tabata Y, Gutta S, Langer R. Controlled delivery Systems for Proteins Using Polyanhydride Microspheres. Pharmaceutical Research An Official Journal of American Associate Pharmacy Science. 1993;**10**:487-496

[33] Joshi A. Microparticulates for ophthalmic drug delivery. Journal of Ocular Pharmacology. 1994;**10**: 29-45

[34] Jang WD, Nakagishi Y, Nishiyama N, Kawauchi S, Morimoto Y, Kikuchi M, et al. Polyion complex micelles for photodynamic therapy: Incorporation of dendritic photosensitizer excitable at long wavelength relevant to improved tissue-penetrating property. Journal of Controlled Release. 2006;**113**:73-79

[35] Usui T, Sugisaki K, Amano S, Jang WD, Nishiyama N, Kataoka K. New drug delivery for corneal neovascularization using polyion complex micelles. Cornea. 2005;**24**:39-42

[36] Ideta R, Tasaka F, Jang WD, Nishiyama N, Zhang GD, Harada A, et al. Nanotechnology-based photodynamic therapy for neovascular disease using a supramolecular nanocarrier loaded with a dendritic photosensitizer. Nano Letters. 2005;**5**:2426-2431

[37] Rajasekaran A, Sivakumar V, Karthika K, Preetha JP, Abirami T. Design and evaluation of polymeric controlled release Natamycin ocular inserts. Kathmandu University Journal of Science, Engineering and Technology. 1970;**6**:108-115

[38] Sabitha K, Sajeeth CI and Santhi K. Google Scholar [Internet]. 2012. [cited 2022 Mar 26]. Available from: https://scholar.google.co.in/scholar?hl=en&as_sdt=0%2C5&q=+Sabitha%2C+K.%2C+Sajeeth%2C+C.I.+and+Santhi%2C+K.+%282012%29+Chitosan+Nanoparticles%3A+A+Novel+Vehicle+for+the+Enhanced+Ocular+Delivery+of+Moxifloxacin+HCl.+Research+Journal+of+Pharmaceutical%2C+B

[39] Patel H, Patel J, Patel K, Patel R. Ophthalmic drug delivery system-a review. Der Pharmacia Lettre. 2010;**2**(4):100-115 researchgate.net

[40] Singh V, Ahmad R, Heming T. The challenges of ophthalmic drug delivery: A review. International Journal of Drug Discovery. Bioinfo Publications. 2011;**3**:56-62

[41] Kumar KPS. Ocular inserts : A novel controlled drug delivery system. The Pharma Innovation. 2013;**1**:1-14

[42] Gupta D. Review on Ocular Drug Delivery.... - Google Scholar [Internet]. 2011. [cited 2022 Mar 26]. Available from: https://scholar.google.co.in/scholar?hl=en&as_sdt=0%2C5&q=Gupta%2C+D.+%282011%29+Review+on+Ocular+Drug+Delivery.+Dehradun+Institute+of+Technology%2C+Dehradun.+++&btnG=

[43] Almeida H, Amaral MH, Lobão P, Lobo JMS. In situ gelling systems: A strategy to improve the bioavailability of ophthalmic pharmaceutical formulations. Drug Discovery Today. 2014;**19**:400-412

[44] Shah AV, Serajuddin ATM. Development of solid self-emulsifying drug delivery system (SEDDS) I: Use of poloxamer 188 as both solidifying and emulsifying agent for lipids. Pharmaceutical Research. 2012;**29**:2817-2832

[45] Callender SP, Wettig SD. Phase behavior of non-ionic surfactant-medium chain triglyceride-water microemulsion systems. Journal of

Surfactants and Detergents. John Wiley & Sons, Ltd; 2021;24:603-629

[46] Alami-Milani M, Zakeri-Milani P, Valizadeh H, Salehi R, Salatin S, Naderinia A, et al. Novel pentablock copolymers as thermosensitive self-assembling micelles for ocular drug delivery. Advanced Pharmaceutical Bulletin. 2017;**7**:11-20

[47] Cuong N Van, Hsieh MF, Chen YT, Liau I. Synthesis and characterization of PEG-PCL-PEG triblock copolymers as carriers of doxorubicin for the treatment of breast cancer. Journal of Applied Polymer Science. Wiley Periodicals, Inc; 2010;117:3694-3703

[48] Perret R, Skoulios A. Synthèse et caractérisation de copolymères séquencés polyoxyéthylène/poly-ε-caprolactone. Die Makromolekulare Chemie: Macromolecular Chemistry and Physics. 1972;**156**:143-156

[49] Gong CY, Wang YJ, Wang XH, Wei XW, Wu QJ, Wang BL, et al. Biodegradable self-assembled PEG-PCL-PEG micelles for hydrophobic drug delivery, part 2: In vitro and in vivo toxicity evaluation. Journal of Nanoparticle Research. 2011;**13**:721-731

[50] Luo Z, Jin L, Xu L, Zhang ZL, Yu J, Shi S, et al. Thermosensitive PEG-PCL-PEG (PECE) hydrogel as an in situ gelling system for ocular drug delivery of diclofenac sodium. Drug Delivery. Taylor and Francis Ltd. 2016;**23**:63-68

[51] Peng R, Qin G, Li X, Lv H, Qian Z, Yu L. The PEG-PCL-PEG hydrogel as an implanted ophthalmic delivery system after glaucoma filtration surgery; a pilot study. Medical Hypothesis, Discovery and Innovation in Ophthalmology. 2014;**3**:3-8

[52] Sun X, Xu C, Wu G, Ye Q, Wang C. Review poly(lactic-co-glycolic acid): Applications and future prospects for periodontal tissue regeneration. Polymers (Basel). 2017;**9**:189

[53] Mahapatro A, Singh DK. Biodegradable nanoparticles are excellent vehicle for site directed in-vivo delivery of drugs and vaccines. Journal of Nanobiotechnology. 2011;**9**:55

[54] Danhier F, Ansorena E, Silva JM, Coco R, Le Breton A, Préat V. PLGA-based nanoparticles: An overview of biomedical applications. Journal of Controlled Release. 2012;**161**:505-522

[55] Tsai CH, Wang PY, Lin IC, Huang H, Liu GS, Tseng CL. Ocular drug delivery: Role of degradable polymeric nanocarriers for ophthalmic application. International Journal of Molecular Sciences. 2018;**19**:2830

[56] Rigotti A. Absorption, transport, and tissue delivery of vitamin E. Molecular Aspects of Medicine. 2007;**28**:423-436

[57] Sharma PK, Sharma HP, Chakole CM, Pandey J, Chauhan MK. Application of vitamin E TPGS in ocular therapeutics – Attributes beyond excipient. Journal of the Indian Chemical Society. 2022;**99**:1-9

[58] Yang C, Wu T, Qi Y, Zhang Z. Recent advances in the application of vitamin E TPGS for drug delivery. Theranostics. 2018;**8**:464-485

[59] Cholkar K, Gunda S, Earla R, Pal D, Mitra AK. Nanomicellar topical aqueous drop formulation of rapamycin for Back-of-the-eye delivery. AAPS PharmSciTech. Springer New York LLC. 2015;**16**:610-622

[60] Jõhannesson G, Moya-Ortega MD, Ásgrímsdõttir GM, Lund SH, Thorsteinsdõttir M, Loftsson T, et al.

Kinetics of γ-cyclodextrin nanoparticle suspension eye drops in tear fluid. Acta Ophthalmologica. Blackwell Publishing Ltd. 2014;**92**:550-556

[61] Loftsson T, Brewster ME. Pharmaceutical applications of cyclodextrins: Effects on drug permeation through biological membranes. The Journal of Pharmacy and Pharmacology. 2011;**63**:1119-1135

[62] Loftsson T. Drug permeation through biomembranes: Cyclodextrins and the unstirred water layer. Die Pharmazie. 2012;**67**:363-370

[63] Tanito M, Hara K, Takai Y, Matsuoka Y, Nishimura N, Jansook P, et al. Topical dexamethasone-cyclodextrin microparticle eye drops for diabetic macular edema. Investigative Ophthalmology and Visual Science. 2011;**52**:7944-7948

[64] Kaur IP, Kanwar M. Ocular preparations: The formulation approach. Drug Development and Industrial Pharmacy. 2002;**28**:473-493

[65] Kaur I, Chhabra S, Aggarwal D. Role of Cyclodextrins in Ophthalmics. Current Drug Delivery. 2005;**1**: 351-360

[66] Loftsson T, Stefánsson E. Cyclodextrins and topical drug delivery to the anterior and posterior segments of the eye. International Journal of Pharmaceutics. 2017;**531**:413-423

[67] Chaudhari P, Ghate VM, Lewis SA. Supramolecular cyclodextrin complex: Diversity, safety, and applications in ocular therapeutics. Experimental Eye Research. 2019;**189**:1-11

[68] Warren F. Handbook of pharmaceutical excipients. American Journal of Health Pharmacy. 1987;**44**:1946-1948

[69] Amin PD, Bhogte CP, Deshpande MA. Studies on gel tears. Drug Development and Industrial Pharmacy. Taylor & Francis. 1996;**22**:735-739

[70] Lu G. Recent advances in developing ophthalmic formulations: A patent review. Recent Patents on Drug Delivery & Formulation. 2009;**4**:49-57

[71] Treatment of Keratoconjunctivitis Sicca with Lacrimal... - Google Scholar [Internet]. [cited 2022 Mar 28]. Available from: https://scholar.google.co.in/scholar?hl=en&as_sdt=0%2C5&q=+Treatment+of+keratoconjunctivitis+sicca+with+lacrimal+gel%3A+a+multicentre+randomized+study.+J+Fr+Ophtalmol+14%285%29%3A321-6+&btnG=

[72] Johnson ME, Murphy PJ, Boulton M. Carbomer and sodium hyaluronate eyedrops for moderate dry eye treatment. Optometry and Vision Science. 2008;**85**:750-757

[73] Christiansen A, Backensfeld T, Kühn S, Weitschies W. Stability of the non-ionic surfactant polysorbate 80 investigated by HPLC-MS and charged aerosol detector. Die Pharmazie. 2011;**66**:666-671

[74] Tang X, Huston KJ, Larson RG. Molecular dynamics simulations of structure-property relationships of tween 80 surfactants in water and at interfaces. The Journal of Physical Chemistry. B. American Chemical Society. 2014;**118**:12907-12918

[75] Aboumanei MH, Abdelbary AA, Ibrahim IT, Tadros MI, El-Kolaly MT. Design and development of microemulsion systems of a new antineoplaston A10 analog for

enhanced intravenous antitumor activity: In vitro characterization, molecular docking, 125I-radiolabeling and in vivo biodistribution studies. International Journal of Pharmaceutics. 2018;**545**:240-253

[76] Strickley RG. Solubilizing excipients in Oral and injectable formulations. Pharmaceutical Research. 2004;**21**:201-230

[77] Nayak K, Misra M. A review on recent drug delivery systems for posterior segment of eye. Biomedicine & Pharmacotherapy. Elsevier. 2018;**107**:1564-1582

Section 3

Pharmacokinetics and Metabolism

Chapter 6

Interplay between Pharmacokinetics and Pharmacogenomics

Alaa Yehya

Abstract

Pharmacogenomics represents an attempt to optimize the efficacy of drugs, minimize adverse drug reactions, and facilitate drug discovery, development, and approval. Understanding an individual's genetic makeup can be the key to creating personalized drugs with greater efficacy and safety, as pharmacogenetic testing can be used to identify individuals who may be more susceptible to adverse drug reactions. Interindividual variability in the pharmacokinetics of many medicinal products is prone to interindividual variability. Pharmacogenomics should be considered one of the factors affecting the pharmacokinetics of a drug. When a polymorphism in a metabolizing enzyme and/or transporter causes a difference in exposure, it may alter efficacy or safety.

Keywords: pharmacogenomics, pharmacokinetics, pharmacology, drug, genetic testing

1. Introduction

Pharmacogenetics is a component of precision medicine in which patient-specific genes are used to optimize the medical care of patients, which serves to achieve an optimal drug response in terms of efficacy and toxicity [1]. Observations related to the dependence of drug effects on the genetic constitution of the recipient can be traced back to the 1950s, when reports of primaquine-caused hemolysis were seen in individuals who were glucose-6-phosphate (G6PD)-deficient [2]. Researchers examined why different people had such diverse responses to the same medication. In 1957, Arno Motulsky, a pioneer of medical genetics, published a paper titled "Drug Reactions, Enzymes, and Biochemical Genetics." Freidrich Vogel, a German geneticist, is credited with coining the term "pharmacogenetics" in 1959 to explain the influence of inherited genetic characteristics on clinical responses to xenobiotics. Werner Kalow, a German clinical pharmacologist, created the framework of pharmacogenetics in his book *Pharmacogenetics: Heredity and Drug Response*, which collected known research at the time, including his personal findings on genetic variation and ethnicity [3].

Between 1977 and 1988, an increasing number of different genetic variants and their corresponding enzymatic functions were reported [4]. In 1999, the National Institutes of Health (NIH) announced a mission "to enable the formation of a series of multi-disciplinary research groups funded to conduct studies addressing research problems in pharmacogenetics" [5]. The Pharmacogenetics Research Network (PGRN) was created in 2000, with a mission "to catalyze and lead research in precision medicine for the discovery and translation of genomic variation influencing therapeutic and adverse drug effects" [6]. In the same year, the Pharmacogenomics Knowledge Base (PharmGKB) was released, which is a searchable referenced database of clinically actionable gene-drug associations and the relationships between genotypes and their produced phenotypes [7].

Reports focused on specific genes have been implicated in medication response for many years; single-nucleotide polymorphisms (SNPs) are the most frequently encountered genetic variants. High-density maps of SNPs also make them the most technically accessible class of genetic variants. By correlating SNPs and drug response data, one will have gained an ability to predict drug efficacy or toxicity within reasonable limits for any individual [8]. With the completion of the human genome sequencing project in 2001, a cutting-edge information technology capable of processing tens of thousands of raw sequence data became accessible [9]. Several population-based programs were launched in subsequent years. The term "pharmacogenomics" has emerged to refer to a better knowledge of the influence genetic diversity has, in many genes, on medication pharmacology. Currently, research institutes, companies, and government laboratories are rapidly moving on toward acquiring pharmacogenomic database management systems (DBMS), which are meant to combine public and proprietary genomic databases, clinical data sets, and results from high-throughput screening technologies [10].

Drug safety is the evaluation and study of the pharmacological effects of a potential drug that are unrelated to the desired therapeutic effect [11]. It is an essential element throughout the spectrum of drug discovery and development. A focus on variation related to genes involved in a drug's pharmacokinetics (PK), which is the complex interplay of absorption, distribution, metabolism, and excretion, can be helpful for the prevention and treatment of patients experiencing with adverse drug reaction (ADR) [12]. Consequently, it can assist in choosing the appropriate and safe drug and dosage for each patient [13]. The term "population pharmacokinetic" (PPK) was first used by Sheiner in 1977 for investigating the typical PK of a drug in a large target population using available data. The PPK approach aims to quantitate the effects of various physiologic factors on drug PK with the overall goal of explaining as much variability as possible [14]. Mathematical models are developed to estimate the population-specific pharmacokinetic model parameters for a given drug. For example, parameters can be used to quantify the relationship, e.g., of clearance to individual physiology, such as the function of the liver, kidney, or heart [15]. A dose regimen can then be adjusted to achieve a specific clinical goal, such as drug exposure, within the therapeutic concentration window in the whole population or, if necessary, for special subpopulations characterized by their individual physiology. It must be considered that the significant variability of genetic information is transmitted from one generation to the other and is not always unaltered, creating a further degree of variability with great potential clinical relevance [16]. Pharmacogenomics accounts for ≈80% of the variability in drug efficacy and safety. Over 400 genes are clinically relevant in drug metabolism, and ≈200 pharmagenes are associated ADRs. The main role of pharmacogenetics is to translate genetic information into everyday clinical practice and lower the impact of ADRs, both for patients and for the healthcare system. The Food and Drug Administration (FDA) recently approved a safety labeling change for multiple drugs, guiding clinicians to identify individuals who may be "more susceptible" to ADR [17]. This labeling change does not constitute a requirement for testing prior to drug use but represents a step toward the establishment of such testing as a standard of practice.

The development of diagnostic tests for clinically significant disorders should be the emphasis of pharmacogenomics research [18]. Not every association results in a potentially valuable pharmacogenetic test, and financial and technological resources may be squandered if the significance of more easily quantifiable values is not initially ruled out [19]. For example, 5-hydroxytryptamine-3 receptor antagonists, which are used to treat nausea and vomiting, are known to be metabolized by the cytochrome P450 2D6 (CYP2D6) enzyme. Kim et al. discovered genotype-dependent pharmacokinetics for tropisetron in healthy volunteers [20], indicating that cancer patients who are ultrarapid metabolizers (UM) are undertreated by a standard dose of tropisetron. This idea was tested in 270 cancer patients by Kaiser and colleagues. There were more nausea and vomiting episodes in patients with a significant number of functioning CYP2D6 alleles. Patients given 4 mg of ondansetron to prevent postoperative nausea and vomiting had a similar outcome [21]. The impact of the UM phenotype on the pharmacokinetics and therapeutic efficacy of 5-hydroxytryptamine 3 receptor antagonists is clearly demonstrated by these studies. The "number needed to genotype" (i.e., the number of individuals needed to genotype to prevent one patient from experiencing needless nausea and vomiting) appeared to be 50 due to the low frequency of the UM genotype in persons of northern European origin [22]. This number is likely too high to incorporate pharmacogenetic testing into normal clinical practice and, more significantly, simpler options for preventing nausea, such as dosage titration or the use of an alternate antiemetic regimen, are currently available [23].

The molecular biology background of pharmacogenetics describes variations seen in drugs' pharmacokinetic phases and/or pharmacodynamics, where drug receptors and other targets may be different from one patient to another [24]. This chapter focuses on the interplay between pharmacokinetics and pharmacogenomics.

2. Single-gene pharmacokinetics disorders

2.1 Pseudocholinesterase deficiency

Pseudocholinesterase is a plasma enzyme produced in the liver that is responsible for the metabolism of common muscle relaxants, including succinylcholine and mivacurium [25]. The inherited form of the enzyme transfers in an autosomal recessive manner. Patients with defective inherited forms of pseudocholinesterase (heterozygotes and homozygotes) present with prolonged muscular paralysis. Acquired pseudocholinesterase deficiency can develop in a variety of diseases or as a side effect of certain medications [26]. Pseudocholinesterase deficiency can be induced by malnutrition, pregnancy and the postpartum period, burns, liver illness, renal disease, cancer, infections, and medications such as steroids and cytotoxic agents [27]. Both acquired and hereditary defects are considered uncommon. Caucasian males of European origin, as well as Alaskan Native tribes, have the highest frequency of pseudocholinesterase deficiency [28]. In pseudocholinesterase-deficient patients, there is no particular therapy for neuromuscular paralysis; nevertheless, respiratory assistance with mechanical ventilation can be provided until the neuromuscular blockade is resolved [29]. Nondepolarizing neuromuscular blockers, such as atracurium, rocuronium, and vecuronium, are indicated for those with pseudocholinesterase deficiency. In addition, relatives of those who have been diagnosed with pseudocholinesterase deficiency are advised to get tested for the condition [30].

2.2 Acute intermittent porphyria

Acute intermittent porphyria (AIP) is a pharmacogenetic disease caused by a porphyrin metabolic defect characterized by a lack of porphobilinogen deaminase and a rise in the activity of delta-aminolevulinic acid synthase—two essential enzymes required for heme production [31]. Patients may have stomach discomfort, vomiting, muscular weakness, constipation, and neuropsychiatric symptoms during an episode. Clinical episodes are produced by many drugs (including barbiturates, antiseizure drugs, and sulfonamide antibiotics), hormones, and dietary variables, all of which induce hepatic delta-aminolevulinic acid synthase [32].

The most accurate approach for confirming AIP in patients and their symptom-free relatives is DNA analysis. The hydroxymethylbilane synthase (HMBS) gene is directly sequenced to discover a mutation in the proband as well as asymptomatic gene carriers among family members [33]. The sensitivity of the mutation analysis ranges from 90–100%. So far, 391 mutations in the HMBS gene have been reported. Thus, DNA testing in a family's index case may be more difficult and time-consuming, but mutation analysis thereafter may quickly identify numerous family members at risk [34].

Heme infusions are frequently used to reduce the intensity and frequency of recurring episodes. The goal of this treatment is to significantly lower the level of porphyrin precursors in the blood. Most individuals react effectively, although long-term therapy may lead to exogenic heme dependency. As a result, a patient's heme need may grow from monthly to twice-weekly infusions, making treatment discontinuation difficult due to significant porphyric symptoms. The use of heme preparations on a regular basis might cause thrombotic problems in the superficial veins, necessitating the use of a permanent central venous catheter [35]. Furthermore, long-term heme therapy might result in iron excess and hemosiderosis, which can cause organ damage. Hepatopathy, heart failure and endocrinopathies may arise as a result of the disease progressing. Iron burden in organs is shown by computed tomography (CT) or magnetic resonance imaging (MRI) [36]. Venesections are generally unpopular, although iron chelates can help. Preventative actions can be taken if family members are tested to determine whether they are genetic carriers. Symptomatic treatment, a high carbohydrate diet, and intravenous hematin injection are all used to treat attacks [37].

2.3 Drug acetylation deficiency

N-acetyl transferase (NATS) activities in human hepatic drug metabolizing enzymes have previously been identified as a source of inter-individual heterogeneity in drug metabolism [38]. The liver's cytochrome P450 enzymes are primarily responsible for phase I oxidation, whereas phase 2 conjugations include glucuronidation, sulfation, and acetylation [39]. Two genes (NAT 1) and (NAT 2) are now known to control N-acetyl transferase (NAT), with NAT 2 A and B accounting for clinically significant metabolic variance [40].

Caffeine, isoniazid, nitrazepam, and sulfonamides are among the many common medications that are acetylated. Aromatic and heterocyclic amines are also carcinogenic, which has led to the theory that NAT genotypes are linked to cancer risk. Individuals can be divided into two groups after receiving sulfamethazine, caffeine, or another marker drug and having plasma and urine drug concentrations measured after a standard time interval: fast acetylators with only low concentrations of the parent drug remaining in the blood and slow acetylators with much higher concentrations of the parent drug remaining in the blood [41]. The frequency of fast and slow acetylators varies by ethnicity; Caucasian and Negro populations have almost equal numbers of fast and slow acetylators, whereas Oriental races have over 90% quick acetylators. The slow acetylator phenotype predominates among Arab people in Asia (e.g., Saudi Arabia and the United Arab Emirate) [42, 43] and North Africa (e.g., Egypt and Morocco) [40, 44].

3. Genetic variants affecting pharmacokinetics

Genetic variation in drug-metabolizing enzymes and/or drug transporter genes might impact drug exposure in terms of PK key parameters, such as maximum drug concentration (Cmax) and area under the curve (AUC) [45]. These differences can affect a patient's loading dose, maintenance dose, dosing interval, and as a result, medication response and safety [46, 47].

3.1 Pharmacogenomics of drug-metabolizing enzymes

In the last decade, technical advancements in gene scanning and gene variant identification have substantially increased our understanding of the function of pharmacogenetics in drug metabolism [48, 49]. The number of genetic variants identified for genes coding for drug-metabolizing enzymes (DMEs) considerably increased in the early 2000s and continues to increase. Variation in drug metabolism and drug response can be caused by temporary factors, such as transient enzyme inhibition and induction, or by permanent causes, such as genetic mutation, gene deletion, or amplification among people of the same body weight and on the same medicine dosage. However, not all variants result in significant changes in enzyme activity. Genetic polymorphism can be associated with three phenotype classes based on drug metabolizing ability: the extensive drug metabolizer phenotype (EM) is found in the general population; the poor drug metabolizer phenotype (PM) is caused by mutation and/or deletion of both alleles and is linked to the accumulation of specific drug substrates; and gene amplification causes the UM phenotype, which results in increased drug metabolism [50]. The cytochrome P450 enzymes in families 1–3 mediate 70–90% of all phase I-dependent metabolism of available drugs [51]. The polymorphic forms of P450s are responsible for the development of approximately 86% of the reported adverse drug reactions (ADRs) of substrate drugs. Polymorphic enzymes (in particular, CYP2C9, CYP2C19, and CYP2D6) mediate around 40% of P450-mediated drug metabolism [52]. The major CYP450 forms that are important in human drug metabolism are shown in **Table 1**, together with their main substrates and the clinical consequences of the polymorphism.

3.2 Pharmacogenomics of drug transporters

The distribution of drug transporters in tissues key to pharmacokinetics, such as the intestine (absorption), blood-brain barrier (distribution), liver (metabolism), and kidneys (excretion), strongly suggests that genetic variation associated with changes in protein expression or function of these transporters may have a substantial impact on systemic drug exposure and toxicity [53]. In the last decade, a greater focus has been given to the impact of genetic variation in membrane transporters on the pharmacokinetics and toxicity of numerous therapeutic drugs [54]. While most transporter-related pharmacogenetic research has been related to classic genes

Metabolizing enzyme	Example substrates	Major allelic variants	Clinical consequence of the polymorphism	Ref
CYP2D6	Atomoxetine, propranolol, tramadol	CYP2D6*4 CYP2D6*10 CYP2D6*17 CYP2D6*41	Altered drug dosage	[47]
CYP1A2	Caffeine, duloxetine, melatonin, clozapine	CYP1A2*1 K	Reduced enzyme inducibility	[48]
CYP2C9	Celecoxib, glimepiride, phenytoin, warfarin	CYP2C9*2 CYP2C9*3	Altered drug dosage	[49]
CYP2C19	Omeprazole, diazepam, rabeprazole, voriconazole	CYP2C19*2 CYP2C19*3	Altered drug dosage	[50]

Table 1.
CYP450 enzymes and related polymorphisms.

Drug transporter	Example substrates	Polymorphism	Clinical consequence	Ref
OATP1B1	Atorvastatin, pravastatin, repaglinide, methotrexate	SLCO1B1*5 Val174Ala c.521 T > C	Increased susceptibility to drug induced adverse events	[54]
ABCG2	Sulfasalazine, atorvastatin	(rs2231142 Gln141Lys c.421C > A	Increased susceptibility to drug induced adverse events	[55]
OCT1	Metformin, cisplatin	R61C P160L G401S G465R	Altered drug dosage	[56]
ABCB1	Irinotecan, mycophenalic acid	3435C > T 2677G/T/A	Increased susceptibility to drug induced adverse events	[57]
SLC6A4	Citalopram, respiridone	5-HTTLPR	Altered drug response	[58]

Table 2.
Drug transporters and related polymorphisms.

encoding the outward-directed ATP-binding cassette (ABC) transporters, such as ABCB1 (P-glycoprotein), ABCC2 (MRP2), and ABCG2 (BCRP), more studies have been conducted in recent years evaluating genes encoding solute carriers (SLC) that mediate the cellular uptake of drugs, such as SLCO1B1 (OATP1B1) and SLC22A1 (OCT1) [55]. The main drug transporters are shown in **Table 2**, together with their main substrates and the clinical consequences of the polymorphism(s).

4. Utility of pharmacogenomics and clinically available tests

One of the earliest uses of sequencing the human genome was expected to be clinical testing to predict medication response. New pharmacogenetic tests have a positive or substantial impact on prescription practice, such as the adoption of a different medication or dosage regimen, which results in quantifiable improvements in patient outcomes [56]. Despite the availability of tests, several barriers have hindered their implementation in ordinary clinical practice, including poor knowledge among health-care professionals, ethical concerns, and the cost-effectiveness of the clinical outcome [57]. Furthermore, determining medication responses in complex multifactorial characteristics is difficult due to the interaction of many genes and genetic variations with environmental variables, and the genetic element may only have a minor influence on the outcome of treatment [58]. Much of the early published research focused on single pathogenic mutations that are particularly conspicuous or that have an obvious or unambiguous "all or nothing" therapy [59]. In fact, the likelihood of medication benefit and risk is frequently a continuum with a broad range of variance among individuals in a community, and relying on a single predictive biomarker to guide the treatment of serious diseases may not be accurate or reliable enough. Confirming analytic validity (test accuracy and reliability) and determining clinical utility should be the first steps in assessing pharmacogenetic indicators in clinical treatment [60]. There are additional health-economic issues to address, such as whether the genetic markers are common enough in their patient population to warrant the screening expenses [61]. The practicality of applying the biomarker testing method in a way that does not delay patient care will then be examined by policymakers and funding agencies. When compared with the current availability of preemptive testing for many genetic markers, the previous practice of single gene as needed, or "one at a time'" testing, might appear inefficient and costly [60]. Several obstacles to pharmacogenomics implementation have been identified and reported in the literature. Many of these issues are comparable with those that arise when introducing any new therapeutic service in a variety of practice settings. Securing administrative and provider buy-in, building effective physician relationships, and integrating a new service into an established clinical workflow are just a few of the common obstacles [62]. Still, fast testing utilizing multi-gene panels is becoming more widely available; an individual's genetic data from a single sample may now be used to advise them about a variety of treatment options that may occur later in their lives.

4.1 Warfarin and CYP2C9/VKCOR

The most commonly prescribed medication for which a pharmacogenetic test has been proposed is warfarin [63]. The adoption of such testing as a standard of care has had to overcome three major challenges: (i) the presence of an alternative biomarker, the international normalized ratio, which is widely used and trusted by the practice community [64]; (ii) the need for specific dosing guidelines resulting from testing; and (iii) the need to demonstrate improvements not only in short-term toxicity but also in long-term toxicity [65]. Several dosage algorithms have been presented, and an international collaboration of researchers led by the PharmGKB (Pharmacogenomics Knowledge Base) has developed a clear, generalizable dosing methodology. Only the VKORC1 (P = 6.2 10–13) and CYP2C9 (P = 5 10–4) polymorphisms were found to be significant in a genome-wide association investigation of about 550,000 polymorphisms, suggesting that extensive and expensive trials would be necessary to find other relevant genetic variations [66]. The United States Food and Drug Administration (FDA) has revised the labeling to include genetic information, recognizing the importance of the relationship between the CYP2C9 genotype and the risk of severe bleeding episodes as well as a number of effectiveness surrogates [67]. Additional studies on the specificity and sensitivity of testing for both effectiveness and toxicity will likely be required before existing practice guidelines are amended to incorporate CYP2C9 9 and VKORC1 testing as clinical recommendations [68].

4.2 Tamoxifen and CYP2D6

Numerous studies across the world have investigated correlations between genotype and clinical outcome since the Consortium on Breast Cancer Pharmacogenomics identified a substantial relationship between the active metabolite endoxifen concentrations and the CYP2D6 genotype [69, 70]. Although more than 10 studies have been published on the subject, they are all small, and none of the large prospective trials comparing tamoxifen to aromatase inhibitors have been opened for analysis [71]. This is important, since the publishing of small studies might lead to selection bias and underpowered results in the research. Given that complex CYP genotypes can now be determined from paraffin sections [72], these data should be critical to the long-term clinical utility of CYP2D6 testing for tamoxifen efficacy in the many practice settings where it is used.

4.3 (5-fluorouracil) and dihydropyrimidine dehydrogenase deficiency

5-Fluorouracil is a chemotherapeutic medication commonly used to treat solid tumors, but its inconsistent effectiveness is exacerbated by its equally variable and often severe mucocutaneous toxicity [73]. The main metabolic enzyme in the target of 5-fluorouracil, dihydropyrimidine dehydrogenase, has a significant number of functional genetic variations [74]. Because testing for these variations cannot identify all cases of toxicity, their specificity and sensitivity are limited. This might be due to contributions from unknown genetic variations or nongenetic variables, such as age and gender, which have been shown to impact 5-fluorouracil clearance and toxicity [75]. Genome-wide association studies and the development of predictive scores integrating both clinical and genetic variables may be useful in this regard.

4.4 Irinotecan and UGT1A1

Variable effectiveness and possibly life-threatening toxicity limit the use of irinotecan as an effective therapy for colorectal and lung cancer [76]. Irinotecan is metabolized to the active metabolite SN-38, which is then removed by uridine diphosphate glucuronosyltransferase 1A1 (UGT1A1)-catalyzed phase II glucuronidation [77]. It was immediately realized that this enzyme is also the primary cause of Gilbert's syndrome's benign, congenital hyperbilirubinemia. UGT1A1 polymorphisms are also predictive of irinotecan pharmacokinetics and treatment results, according to a number of studies [78, 79]. Irinotecan's FDA-approved label has been updated to contain a reference to UGT1A1 genetic testing but no precise dosage recommendations. This, along with evidence that UGT1A1 testing may not be predictive for all irinotecan dosage regimens, has limited the test's utility [58]. FDA labeling has not resulted in widespread usage of this test. This might be due to the absence of well-established alternative therapy options for patients with certain UGT1A1 genotypes as well as the unknown effects of testing.

4.5 Azathioprine, 6-mercaptopurine, and thiopurine methyltransferase

Granulocytopenia is a rare but life-threatening complication caused by giving standard dosages of azathioprine or 6-mercaptopurine to those who have homozygous thiopurine methyltransferase gene variations (TPMT) [80]. Although these medicines are approved for the treatment of leukemia in children, most of their clinical usage is in the treatment of inflammatory bowel disease in adults, where there have been fewer studies evaluating their efficacy. The perception that alternative indicators, such as a simple measurement of white blood cell count, may be used in place of the genetic test has limited its usage [81]. Furthermore, the availability of an equally predictive alternative—the test for phenotypic enzyme activity—has led to the increased adoption of this phenotypic test in some situations. The TPMT genotyping test is now included on the FDA labels for the medicines in question, but neither the criteria for testing nor the ramifications of the test's results are specified [82]. Overall, the rarity of the variant phenotype, the availability of alternative predictors, and an FDA label that is neither specific nor proscriptive restrict the widespread utility of testing for the TPMT genotype.

4.6 Abacavir and HLA*B5701

Abacavir's usage in the treatment of HIV/AIDS is linked to severe skin sensitivity, which has severely restricted its use [83]. Fortunately, significant skin responses are strongly linked to a germline HLA variation, and HLA*B5701 testing has been routinely utilized to prevent these reactions all over the world [84]. As a result, the medication is now used more effectively, and genetic testing is now the standard of care when abacavir is administered. The release of large prospective clinical trials demonstrating decreases in the incidence of skin sensitivity responses with clinically acceptable specificity and sensitivity has contributed to this accomplishment [85]. These studies were linked to a significant rise in the usage of testing [86]. However, abacavir is not extensively utilized in all clinical settings, and a single pharmacoeconomic analysis found that HLA-B*5701 testing would remain the favored approach only if abacavir-based treatment was as effective as tenofovir-based treatment and if the cost was lower per month.

4.7 Carbamazepine and HLA-B*1502

Carbamazepine can induce severe skin responses, such as Stevens-Johnson syndrome and toxic epidermal necrolysis, similar to abacavir. These negative occurrences have been linked to a specific HLA allele, HLA-B*1502,18, which is found nearly exclusively in Asian people [87]. HLA-B*1502 genetic testing is available, and the FDA has determined that Asian individuals should be tested before commencing carbamazepine medication [88]. Unless the predicted benefit clearly justifies a higher risk of severe skin responses, carbamazepine should not be initiated if they test positive. Even if a pharmacogenetic impact is limited to a particular ethnic group, rapid FDA action is conceivable when the link is convincing and a therapeutic change may be achieved, as in the instance of carbamazepine. It is worth noting that the identical genetic variation has recently been linked to phenytoin hypersensitivity responses.

4.8 Clozapine and HLA-DQB1

Agranulocytosis, the most serious side effect of clozapine, has been linked to the HLA locus, limiting the use of this essential and effective medicine [89]. An association between the incidence of clozapine-related agranulocytosis and HLA-DQB1*0201 in schizophrenia patients has been reported [90]. This assumption is based on short trials with a small number of 50 patients, making it less powerful and specific than in the instances of abacavir and carbamazepine. As a result, the test has a lower acceptance rate, and recommendations have yet to be developed.

5. Conclusions

The discipline of pharmacogenomics (PGX) has rapidly developed, and its application to patient care is continuing to unfold. It is acknowledged that pharmacogenetics may not be equally important for every drug. Genetic factors influencing drugs' pharmacokinetic phases are centered on drug metabolism and transportation. Pharmacogenetic testing investigations should be promoted in sectors where there is a high probability of a clinically meaningful impact on clinical practice.

Acknowledgements

The seed for this chapter was planted during the author's participation in the Fulbright Program at University of Nebraska Medical Center (UNMC) in the summer of 2021. Special thanks to Dr. Amy Pick for her support, exchange of ideas, and the unique opportunity to wonder.

Conflict of interest

The author declares no conflicts of interest.

Author details

Alaa Yehya
Faculty of Pharmacy, Department of Clinical Pharmacy and Pharmacy Practice, Yarmouk University, Irbid, Jordan

*Address all correspondence to: alaa.yehya@yu.edu.jo

References

[1] Daly AK. Pharmacogenetics: A general review on progress to date. British Medical Bulletin. 2017;**124**(1):65-79

[2] Watson J, Taylor WR, Menard D, Kheng S, White NJ. Modelling primaquine-induced haemolysis in G6PD deficiency. eLife. 2017;**6**:e23061

[3] Kalow W. Pharmacogenomics: Historical perspective and current status. Methods in Molecular Biology. 2005;**311**:3-15

[4] Sosnay PR, Cutting GR. Interpretation of genetic variants. Thorax. 2014;**69**(3):295-297

[5] Ganguly NK, Bano R, Seth SD. Human genome project: Pharmacogenomics and drug development. Indian Journal of Experimental Biology. 2001;**39**(10):955-961

[6] Shuldiner A, Relling M, Peterson J, et al. The pharmacogenomics research network translational pharmacogenetics program: Overcoming challenges of real-world implementation. Clinical Pharmacology & Therapeutics. 2013;**94**(2):207-210

[7] Barbarino JM, Whirl-Carrillo M, Altman RB, Klein TE. PharmGKB: A worldwide resource for pharmacogenomic information. Wiley Interdisciplinary Reviews. Systems Biology and Medicine. 2018;**10**(4):e1417

[8] Alwi ZB. The use of SNPs in pharmacogenomics studies. Malaysian Journal of Medical Sciences. 2005;**12**(2):4-12

[9] Bhasker CR, Hardiman G. Advances in pharmacogenomics technologies. Pharmacogenomics. 2010;**11**(4):481-485

[10] Reischl J, Schroder M, Luttenberger N, et al. Pharmacogenetic research and data protection--challenges and solutions. The Pharmacogenomics Journal. 2006;**6**(4):225-233

[11] Alshammari TM. Drug safety: The concept, inception and its importance in patients' health. Saudi Pharmaceutical Journal. 2016;**24**(4):405-412

[12] Wang K, Weng Z, Sun L, et al. Systematic drug safety evaluation based on public genomic expression (connectivity map) data: Myocardial and infectious adverse reactions as application cases. Biochemical and Biophysical Research Communications. 2015;**457**(3):249-255

[13] Kalinin AA, Higgins GA, Reamaroon N, et al. Deep learning in pharmacogenomics: From gene regulation to patient stratification. Pharmacogenomics. 2018;**19**(7):629-650

[14] Sherwin CM, Kiang TK, Spigarelli MG, Ensom MH. Fundamentals of population pharmacokinetic modelling: Validation methods. Clinical Pharmacokinetics. 2012;**51**(9):573-590

[15] Chow AT, Earp JC, Gupta M, et al. Utility of population pharmacokinetic modeling in the assessment of therapeutic protein-drug interactions. Journal of Clinical Pharmacology. 2014;**54**(5):593-601

[16] Lee PI. Design and power of a population pharmacokinetic study. Pharmaceutical Research. 2001;**18**(1):75-82

[17] Mehta D, Uber R, Ingle T, et al. Study of pharmacogenomic information in FDA-approved drug labeling to facilitate application of precision medicine. Drug Discovery Today. 2020;**25**(5):813-820

[18] Wu AC, Mazor KM, Ceccarelli R, Loomer S, CYJJoPM L.

The implementation process for pharmacogenomic testing for cancer-targeted therapies. Therapies. Journal of personalized medicine. 2018;**8**(4):32

[19] Maitland ML, DiRienzo A, Ratain MJ. Interpreting disparate responses to cancer therapy: The role of human population genetics. Journal of Clinical Oncology. 2006;**24**(14):2151-2157

[20] Kim MK, Cho JY, Lim HS, et al. Effect of the CYP2D6 genotype on the pharmacokinetics of tropisetron in healthy Korean subjects. European Journal of Clinical Pharmacology. 2003;**59**(2):111-116

[21] Kaiser R, Sezer O, Papies A, et al. Patient-tailored antiemetic treatment with 5-hydroxytryptamine type 3 receptor antagonists according to cytochrome P-450 2D6 genotypes. Journal of Clinical Oncology. 2002;**20**(12):2805-2811

[22] Candiotti KA, Birnbach DJ, Lubarsky DA, et al. The impact of pharmacogenomics on postoperative nausea and vomiting: Do CYP2D6 allele copy number and polymorphisms affect the success or failure of ondansetron prophylaxis? Anesthesiology. 2005;**102**(3):543-549

[23] McLeod HL. Genetic strategies to individualize supportive care. Journal of Clinical Oncology. 2002;**20**(12):2765-2767

[24] Di Francia R, Berretta M, Catapano O, Canzoniero LM, LJCc F. Moleculardiagnosticsforpharmacogenomic testing of fluoropyrimidine based-therapy: Costs, methods and applications. Clinical chemistry and laboratory medicine. 2011;**49**(7):1105-1111

[25] Soliday FK, Conley YP, Henker R. Pseudocholinesterase deficiency: A comprehensive review of genetic, acquired, and drug influences. AANA Journal. 2010;**78**(4):313-320

[26] Barta C, Sasvari-Szekely M, Devai A, Kovacs E, Staub M, Enyedi P. Analysis of mutations in the plasma cholinesterase gene of patients with a history of prolonged neuromuscular block during anesthesia. Molecular Genetics and Metabolism. 2001;**74**(4):484-488

[27] Zhang C, Cao H, Wan ZG, Wang J. Prolonged neuromuscular block associated with cholinesterase deficiency. Medicine (Baltimore). 2018;**97**(52):e13714

[28] Zabihi E, Shabanzadeh M, Arabsheibani S, Moghadamnia AA, Baradaran M. Pseudo-cholinesterase polymorphism in Mazandaran province (north of Iran). Caspian Journal of Internal Medicine. 2012;**3**(3):473-477

[29] Whyte AJ, Wang HE. Prehospital airway management complicated by reported pseudocholinesterase deficiency. Prehospital Emergency Care. 2007;**11**(3):343-345

[30] Robles A, Michael M, McCallum R. Pseudocholinesterase deficiency: What the Proceduralist needs to know. The American Journal of the Medical Sciences. 2019;**357**(3):263-267

[31] Stein PE, Badminton MN, Rees DC. Update review of the acute porphyrias. British Journal of Haematology. 2017;**176**(4):527-538

[32] Herrick AL, McColl KE. Acute intermittent porphyria. Best Practice & Research. Clinical Gastroenterology. 2005;**19**(2):235-249

[33] Zhao L, Wang X, Zhang X, et al. Therapeutic strategies for acute intermittent porphyria. Intractable & Rare Diseases Research. 2020;**9**(4):205-216

[34] Ma L, Tian Y, Peng C, Zhang Y, Zhang S. Recent advances in the epidemiology and genetics of acute intermittent porphyria. Intractable & Rare Diseases Research. 2020;**9**(4):196-204

[35] Simon A, Pompilus F, Querbes W, et al. Patient perspective on acute intermittent Porphyria with frequent attacks: A disease with intermittent and chronic manifestations. Patient. 2018;**11**(5):527-537

[36] Stein PE, Badminton MN, Barth JH, et al. Acute intermittent porphyria: Fatal complications of treatment. Clinical Medicine (London, England). 2012;**12**(3):293-294

[37] Baumann K, Kauppinen R. Penetrance and predictive value of genetic screening in acute porphyria. Molecular Genetics and Metabolism. 2020;**130**(1):87-99

[38] Shenfield GM. Genetic polymorphisms, drug metabolism and drug concentrations. The Clinical Biochemist Reviews. 2004;**25**(4):203

[39] Hein DW, Millner LM. Arylamine N-acetyltransferase acetylation polymorphisms: Paradigm for pharmacogenomic-guided therapy-a focused review. Expert Opinion on Drug Metabolism & Toxicology. 2021;**17**(1):9-21

[40] El Desoky ES, AbdelSalam YM, Salama RH, et al. NAT2* 5/* 5 genotype (341T> C) is a potential risk factor for schistosomiasis-associated bladder cancer in Egyptians. Therapeutic Drug Monitoring. 2005;**27**(3):297-304

[41] Pande J, Pande A, Singh S. Acetylator status, drug metabolism and disease. National Medical Journal of India. 2003;**16**(1):24-26

[42] Matar K, Mayet A, Ayoola E, Bawazir S, Al-Faleh F, Al-Wazzan A. Isoniazid acetylation phenotyping in Saudi Arabs. Journal of Clinical Pharmacy and Therapeutics. 2004;**29**(5):443-447

[43] Al-Ahmad MM, Amir N, Dhanasekaran S, et al. Studies on N-acetyltransferase (NAT2) genotype relationships in Emiratis: Confirmation of the existence of phenotype variation among slow Acetylators. Annals of Human Genetics. 2017;**81**(5):190-196

[44] Khassouani C, Hüe B, Jana M, Begaud B, Soulaymani R. Determination of the acetylator phenotype in Moroccan tuberculosis patients using isoniazid as metabolic probe. International Journal of Clinical Pharmacology and Therapeutics. Genetics in Medicine. 2002;**40**(12):548-553

[45] Kozyra M, Ingelman-Sundberg M, VMJGiM L. Rare genetic variants in cellular transporters, metabolic enzymes, and nuclear receptors can be important determinants of interindividual differences in drug response. Genetics in Medicine. 2017;**19**(1):20-29

[46] Woo HI, Kim SR, Huh W, Ko J-W, Lee S-YJD. Association of genetic variations with pharmacokinetics and lipid-lowering response to atorvastatin in healthy Korean subjects. Drug Design, Development and Therapy. 2017;**11**:1135

[47] Athanasiu L, L-LH S, Tesli M, et al. Genome-wide association study identifies common variants associated with pharmacokinetics of psychotropic drugs. Journal of Clinical Psychopharmacology. 2015;**29**(8):884-891

[48] Ingelman-Sundberg M, Rodriguez-Antona C. Pharmacogenetics of drug-metabolizing enzymes: Implications for a safer and more effective drug therapy. Philosophical

Transactions of the Royal Society of London. Series B, Biological Sciences. 2005;**360**(1460):1563-1570

[49] Pinto N, MJCdm ED. Clinically relevant genetic variations in drug metabolizing enzymes. Current Drug Metabolism. 2011;**12**(5):487-497

[50] Roots I, Laschinski G, Arjomand-Nahad F, et al. Genotype and phenotype relationship in drug metabolism. Ernst Schering Research Foundation Workshop. 2007;**59**:81-100

[51] Ingelman-Sundberg M, Oscarson M, McLellan RA. Polymorphic human cytochrome P450 enzymes: An opportunity for individualized drug treatment. Trends in Pharmacological Sciences. 1999;**20**(8):342-349

[52] Finta C, Zaphiropoulos PG. The human cytochrome P450 3A locus. Gene evolution by capture of downstream exons. Gene. 2000;**260**(1-2):13-23

[53] Liang Y, Li S, Chen L. The physiological role of drug transporters. Protein & Cell. 2015;**6**(5):334-350

[54] Roberts AG. The structure and mechanism of drug transporters. Methods in Molecular Biology. 2021;**2342**:193-234

[55] Nigam SK. What do drug transporters really do? Nature Reviews. Drug Discovery. 2015;**14**(1):29-44

[56] Weitzel KW, Duong BQ, Arwood MJ, et al. A stepwise approach to implementing pharmacogenetic testing in the primary care setting. Pharmacogenomics. 2019;**20**(15):1103-1112

[57] de Boer RA, van der Harst P, van Veldhuisen DJ, van den Berg MP. Pharmacogenetics in heart failure: Promises and challenges. Expert Opinion on Pharmacotherapy. 2009;**10**(11):1713-1725

[58] Ikediobi ON, Shin J, Nussbaum RL, et al. Addressing the challenges of the clinical application of pharmacogenetic testing. Clinical Pharmacology & Therapeutics. 2009;**86**(1):28-31

[59] Evans B. Establishing clinical utility of Pharmacogenetic tests in the post-FDAAA era. Clinical Pharmacology & Therapeutics. 2010;**88**(6):749-751

[60] Gillis N, Innocenti F. Evidence required to demonstrate clinical utility of pharmacogenetic testing: The debate continues. Clinical Pharmacology & Therapeutics. 2014;**96**(6):655-657

[61] Amstutz U, Carleton B. Pharmacogenetic testing: Time for clinical practice guidelines. Clinical Pharmacology & Therapeutics. 2011;**89**(6):924-927

[62] Swen JJ, Huizinga TW, Gelderblom H, et al. Translating pharmacogenomics: Challenges on the road to the clinic. PLoS Medicine. 2007;**4**(8):e209

[63] Kamali F, Wynne H. Pharmacogenetics of warfarin. Annual Review of Medicine. 2010;**61**:63-75

[64] Lee MTM, Klein TE. Pharmacogenetics of warfarin: Challenges and opportunities. Journal of Human Genetics. 2013;**58**(6):334-338

[65] Wadelius M, Pirmohamed M. Pharmacogenetics of warfarin: Current status and future challenges. The Pharmacogenomics Journal. 2007;**7**(2):99-111

[66] Cooper GM, Johnson JA, Langaee TY, et al. A genome-wide scan for common genetic variants with a large influence

on warfarin maintenance dose. Blood, The Journal of the American Society of Hematology. 2008;**112**(4):1022-1027

[67] Drozda K, Pacanowski MA, Grimstein C, Zineh I. Pharmacogenetic labeling of FDA-approved drugs: A regulatory retrospective. JACC: Basic to Translational Science. 2018;**3**(4):545-549

[68] Flockhart DA, O'Kane D, Williams MS, et al. Pharmacogenetic testing of CYP2C9 and VKORC1 alleles for warfarin. Genetics in Medicine. 2008;**10**(2):139-150

[69] Dezentjé VO, Opdam FL, Gelderblom H, et al. CYP2D6 genotype- and endoxifen-guided tamoxifen dose escalation increases endoxifen serum concentrations without increasing side effects. Breast Cancer Research and Treatment. 2015;**153**(3):583-590

[70] Madlensky L, Natarajan L, Tchu S, et al. Tamoxifen metabolite concentrations, CYP2D6 genotype, and breast cancer outcomes. Clinical Pharmacology & Therapeutics. 2011;**89**(5):718-725

[71] Lum DW, Perel P, Hingorani AD, Holmes MV. CYP2D6 genotype and tamoxifen response for breast cancer: A systematic review and meta-analysis. PLoS One. 2013;**8**(10):e76648

[72] Rae JM, Cordero KE, Scheys JO, Lippman ME, Flockhart DA, Johnson MD. Genotyping for polymorphic drug metabolizing enzymes from paraffin-embedded and immunohistochemically stained tumor samples. Pharmacogenetics and Genomics. 2003;**13**(8):501-507

[73] Amstutz U, Froehlich TK, Largiadèr CR. Dihydropyrimidine dehydrogenase gene as a major predictor of severe 5-fluorouracil toxicity. Pharmacogenomics. 2011;**12**(9):1321-1336

[74] Morel A, Boisdron-Celle M, Fey L, et al. Clinical relevance of different dihydropyrimidine dehydrogenase gene single nucleotide polymorphisms on 5-fluorouracil tolerance. Molecular Cancer Therapeutics. 2006;**5**(11):2895-2904

[75] Lee AM, Shi Q, Pavey E, et al. DPYD variants as predictors of 5-fluorouracil toxicity in adjuvant colon cancer treatment (NCCTG N0147). Journal of the National Cancer Institute. (JNCI) 2014;**106**(12)

[76] Vallböhmer D, Iqbal S, Yang DY, et al. Molecular determinants of irinotecan efficacy. International Journal of Cancer. 2006;**119**(10):2435-2442

[77] Bai Y, Wu H-w, Ma X, Liu Y, Zhang Y-h. Relationship between UGT1A1* 6/* 28 gene polymorphisms and the efficacy and toxicity of irinotecan-based chemotherapy. OncoTargets and Therapy. 2017;**10**:3071

[78] Han J-Y, Lim H-S, Shin ES, et al. Comprehensive analysis of UGT1A polymorphisms predictive for pharmacokinetics and treatment outcome in patients with non-small-cell lung cancer treated with irinotecan and cisplatin. Journal of Clinical Oncology. 2006;**24**(15):2237

[79] Innocenti F, Undevia SD, Iyer L, et al. Genetic variants in the UDP-glucuronosyltransferase 1A1 gene predict the risk of severe neutropenia of irinotecan. Journal of Clinical Oncology. 2004;**22**(8):1382-1388

[80] Schwab M, Schäffeler E, Marx C, et al. Azathioprine therapy and adverse drug reactions in patients with inflammatory bowel disease: Impact

of thiopurine S-methyltransferase polymorphism. Pharmacogenetics and Genomics. 2002;**12**(6):429-436

[81] Lichtenstein GR. Use of laboratory testing to guide 6-mercaptopurine/ azathioprine therapy. Gastroenterology. 2004;**127**(5):1558-1564

[82] Gearry RB, Barclay ML. Azathioprine and 6-mercaptopurine pharmacogenetics and metabolite monitoring in inflammatory bowel disease. Journal of Gastroenterology and Hepatology. 2005;**20**(8):1149-1157

[83] Hewitt RG. Abacavir hypersensitivity reaction. Clinical Infectious Diseases. 2002;**34**(8):1137-1142

[84] Waters LJ, Mandalia S, Gazzard B, Nelson M. Prospective HLA-B* 5701 screening and abacavir hypersensitivity: A single Centre experience. AIDS. 2007;**21**(18):2533-2534

[85] Saag M, Balu R, Phillips E, et al. High sensitivity of human leukocyte antigen-b* 5701 as a marker for immunologically confirmed abacavir hypersensitivity in white and black patients. Clinical Infectious Diseases. 2008;**46**(7):1111-1118

[86] Lai-Goldman M, Faruki H. Abacavir hypersensitivity: A model system for pharmacogenetic test adoption. Genetics in Medicine. 2008;**10**(12):874-878

[87] Alfirevic A, Jorgensen AL, Williamson PR, Chadwick DW, Park BK, Pirmohamed M. HLA-B locus in Caucasian patients with carbamazepine hypersensitivity. Pharmacogenomics. 2006;**7**(6):813-818

[88] Ferrell PB, McLeod HL. Carbamazepine, HLA-B* 1502 and risk of Stevens–Johnson syndrome and toxic epidermal necrolysis: US FDA recommendations. Pharmacogenomics. 2008;**9**(10):1543-1546

[89] Wiciński M, Węclewicz MM. Clozapine-induced agranulocytosis/ granulocytopenia: Mechanisms and monitoring. Current Opinion in Hematology. 2018;**25**(1):22-28

[90] Goldstein JI, Jarskog LF, Hilliard C, et al. Clozapine-induced agranulocytosis is associated with rare HLA-DQB1 and HLA-B alleles. Nature Communications. 2014;**5**(1):1-9

Chapter 7

In Vitro Drug Metabolism Studies Using Human Liver Microsomes

Siva Nageswara Rao Gajula, Sakina Asgar Vora,
Amol G. Dikundwar and Rajesh Sonti

Abstract

Metabolism of most pharmaceutical drugs occurs in the liver. In drug metabolism, enzymes convert drugs to highly water-soluble metabolites to facilitate excretion from the body. Thus, *in vitro* models for studying drug metabolism usually target hepatocytes or subcellular liver fractions like microsomes, cytosols, or S9 fractions with high concentrations of specific enzymes. The most popular subcellular fraction used during drug discovery tends to be the microsomes, as these are easy to prepare and store, are amenable to high throughput screening, and are a relatively low-cost option. Understanding the metabolic stability and kinetics of glucuronidation of an investigational drug is crucial for predicting the pharmacokinetic parameters that support dosing and dose frequency. This chapter provides detailed information about metabolite profiling, metabolic stability, glucuronidation kinetics, reactive metabolites identification, CYP enzyme inhibition, and general protocols using human liver microsomes.

Keywords: metabolism, metabolite profiling, metabolic stability, glucuronidation, reactive metabolites, drug–drug interaction

1. Introduction

The evolution of a new drug entity proceeds through a preclinical screening stage, during which the pharmacological and toxicological properties are scrutinized [1]. After oral administration, the drug gets absorbed and reaches the liver through the portal circulation for its metabolism. Cytochrome P450 (CYP450) enzymes are responsible for metabolizing most of the drugs in Phase I metabolism. However, flavin-containing monooxygenase (FMO) and enzymatic or nonenzymatic hydrolysis are also involved in the drug's metabolism but to a lesser extent. Phase II metabolism results in the production of metabolites conjugated to different chemical moieties like glucuronide, sulfate, glutathione, glycine, and acetate [2].

In 2016, the U.S. Food and Drug Administration (FDA) issued regulations for determining the safety and evaluation of drug metabolites for their toxicity in nonclinical species. These guidelines also provide a recommendation for identifying and characterizing drug metabolites. *In vivo* clinical metabolism studies involve the screening of biological matrices such as serum, urine, feces, and hair for identification of metabolites, whereas *in vitro* drug metabolism studies using human liver microsomes (HLM), human hepatocytes (either fresh or cryopreserved), and recombinant expression of cytochrome P450 enzymes (supersomes) in determining the human metabolic pathways [3, 4]. Comprehensive studies for Phase I and Phase II metabolism involve extensive HLM and human hepatocytes [5]. HLM helps determine the activity of drug metabolizing enzymes, CYPs and UGTs, present in the liver conveniently and straightforwardly [6, 7]. Further, it offers numerous advantages: high throughput screening, ease of storage, economic, repeatable, and simple usage with higher chances of clinical success [8]. Characterization of drug metabolic properties, assessing metabolic stability, and identifying metabolites are essential in determining the safety and success of clinical development [9].

2. Drug metabolism: a brief background

The concept of drug metabolism emerged around the mid-19th century but flourished in the 20th century [10]. Metabolism of most pharmaceutical drugs occurs in the liver. In drug metabolism, enzymes convert drugs to highly polar metabolites to facilitate excretion from the body. Drug metabolism helps assess the oral bioavailability, elimination half-life, and clearance of the body's drug substance. The deduced parameters help decide the dose adjustment and the drug substance's administration frequency [11]. The drug concentration should always reside within the therapeutic window, i.e., between the minimum effective concentration (MEC) and the maximum safety concentration (MSC), to avoid therapeutic failure and adverse effects [12]. CYPs being abundant in the liver, metabolize the majority of drugs [12]. Furthermore, CYPs regulate the biotransformation of endogenous as well as exogenous compounds [13]. Among all the CYP isoforms, CYP3A4 contributes to the metabolism of more than 50% of the marketed drugs [14, 15].

Drug metabolism reactions are divided into Phase I, Phase II, and Phase III reactions. Phase I reactions result in oxidation, reduction, and hydrolysis. The Phase I enzyme families include the CYP superfamily, flavin-containing monooxygenases (FMO), monoamine oxidases, alcohol or aldehyde dehydrogenases, reductases, esterases, amidases, and epoxide hydrolases. Phase II reactions lead to the addition or conjugation of highly polar groups to the drug molecule after Phase I reactions. Occasionally, direct Phase II reactions occur when susceptible functional groups are present on the molecule without being preceded by Phase I reactions. Common Phase II reactions include glucuronidation, sulphation, methylation, N-acetylation, and glutathione conjugation [16]. Phase III metabolism occurs through the elimination of drug molecules through the efflux pump [12]. The primary objective of drug metabolism is to eliminate the drug from the body by converting the lipophilic centers to hydrophilic centers, thus making them water-soluble for easy elimination through the kidney [17, 18]. Sometimes, metabolism may result in the conversion of a drug into a toxic metabolite. On the contrary, metabolism also converts an inactive drug (prodrug) to its active metabolite for achieving the desired medicinal results [18]. Many metabolites of known drugs like desloratadine (parent drug- loratadine), oxazepam (parent drug- diazepam), and cetirizine (parent drug- hydroxyzine) have been found to possess equivalent or enhanced therapeutic activity than the parent drug [19]. Similarly, the discovery of paracetamol was precious as it replaced the use of phenacetin, a toxic parent moiety. Hence, the metabolite's activity plays a significant part in bioequivalence studies [20].

First-pass metabolism explains metabolism before a drug reaches systemic circulation. This term refers to orally administered drugs that undergo metabolism in the gut or the liver before reaching the systemic circulation. **Figure 1** illustrates the various barriers to the drug reaching systemic circulation by the first-pass metabolism. During the drug discovery and development phases, the drug's metabolic fate should be kept in mind. Several approaches are in use ranging from empirical data-driven approaches to mechanistic models to predict drug metabolism. The empirical data-driven approaches, such as machine learning, involve approximations and assumptions, thereby providing high-speed predictions with low precision. In contrast, the mechanistic models involve quantum mechanics or molecular dynamics for providing significantly high accuracy; however, they consume time and effort [21].

Factors affecting drug metabolism are categorized into inter-individual factors and intra-individual factors [22, 23]. Inter-individual factors such as genetic factors, species differences, health conditions, enzyme induction/inhibition by xenobiotics or environmental factors, nutritional differences, and behavioral and cultural differences vary across individuals. However, they are uniform throughout the life of the organism [22]. Intra-individual factors can change throughout the lifetime, and different

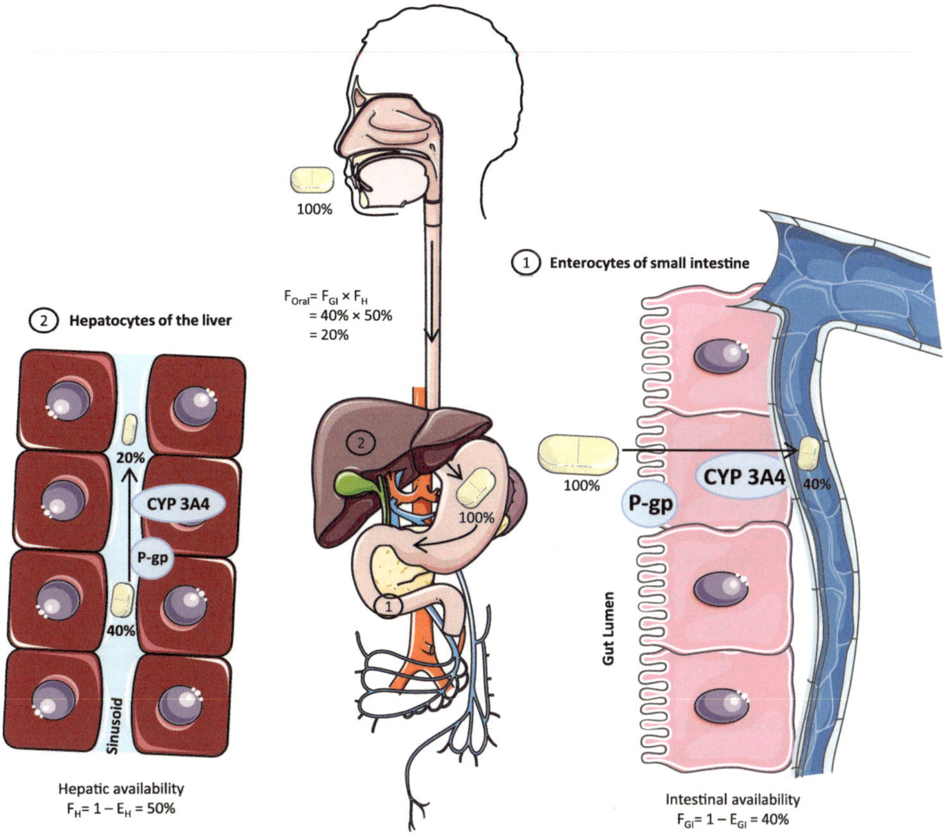

Figure 1.
First-pass metabolism by CYP3A4 and/or transport by P-glycoprotein (P-gp) in the enterocytes of small intestine wall and then hepatocytes of the liver before reaching the systemic circulation. FGI: Intestinal availability, F_H: Hepatic availability,F_{oral}: Oral bioavailability, E_{GI}: Intestinal extraction ratio, E_H: Hepatic extraction ratio.

endogenous and exogenous conditions control these factors, but the effect may be more significant under genetic influence. These can occur through the interaction of xenobiotics with transcription factors or xenobiotics with the drug-metabolizing enzymes. This direct interaction of xenobiotics with the drug-metabolizing enzymes causes the induction or inhibition of those enzymes [23]. Internal factors include age, pregnancy, hormones, sex, diseased state, genetics, and species. In contrast, external factors comprise the environment and diet (alcohol, tobacco, chemicals, and drugs) [24, 25]. Several studies reported that the reduction of rate and efficiency of the drug metabolism in the aging population is due to changes in the drug-metabolizing enzyme activity, variation in plasma protein binding, hepatic blood flow, and decrease in the liver mass, leading to the slowing down of excretion of few metabolized drugs [26]. The results of fasting on drug biotransformation are around 10–20%. This factor becomes crucial when a drug with a narrow therapeutic range is administered or when fasting produces an effect in combination with other factors [27].

In vitro systems help in mimicking and understanding the *in vivo* metabolism process. Of these, liver microsomes and hepatocytes are utilized to predict hepatic clearance [28]. HLM and suspended hepatocytes are the most common *in vitro* methods for determining metabolic stability [29]. They generate metabolites on a large scale for determining metabolic stability and profiling for comparison. The technological advancements have led to the generation of recombinantly expressed CYPs, slicing of the tissues, isolation of hepatocytes, and purification of the enzymes in a reproducible manner [30]. Immobilizing HLM on magnetizable beads coated with silica (HLM-MGBS) showed increased *in-vitro* metabolic efficiency [31]. The cellular or tissue models are used to assess the toxicity of the drug substance and its metabolites in cells or tissues [32, 33]. The placental toxicity of anticancer drugs was elucidated using placental tissue explants and trophoblast cell lines [34].

3. HLM: a best *in vitro* model to conduct high-throughput drug metabolism studies

HLM are the subcellular fractions derived from the liver's endoplasmic reticulum obtained by differential high-speed centrifugation. **Figure 2** displays the steps involved in the preparation of HLM from the human liver. HLM contains various enzymes such as CYPs, flavin-monooxygenase (FMO), carboxylesterases, epoxide hydrolase, and UGTs, making it a preferred *in vitro* model for drug metabolism studies. Assessing interindividual variability is possible with HLM as the activity of the microsomes differs in different individuals. This interindividual variability can be minimized while performing general metabolism studies by pooling the microsomes from different individuals. Microsomes from other human organs (intestine, kidney, lung) are also available and are utilized to evaluate extra-hepatic metabolism [35]. HLM aids in various studies like metabolite identification and profiling, assessment of interspecies variations, estimation of *in vivo* clearance, reaction phenotyping, and elucidation of the metabolic pathways [5, 8, 30, 36–38]. Furthermore, gender-specific microsomes are utilized in studying gender-based disparities in drug metabolism studies.

NADPH or NADPH regenerating system (NRS) is essential for the incubation process, and while determining the UGT activity, UDGPA and alamethicin are the

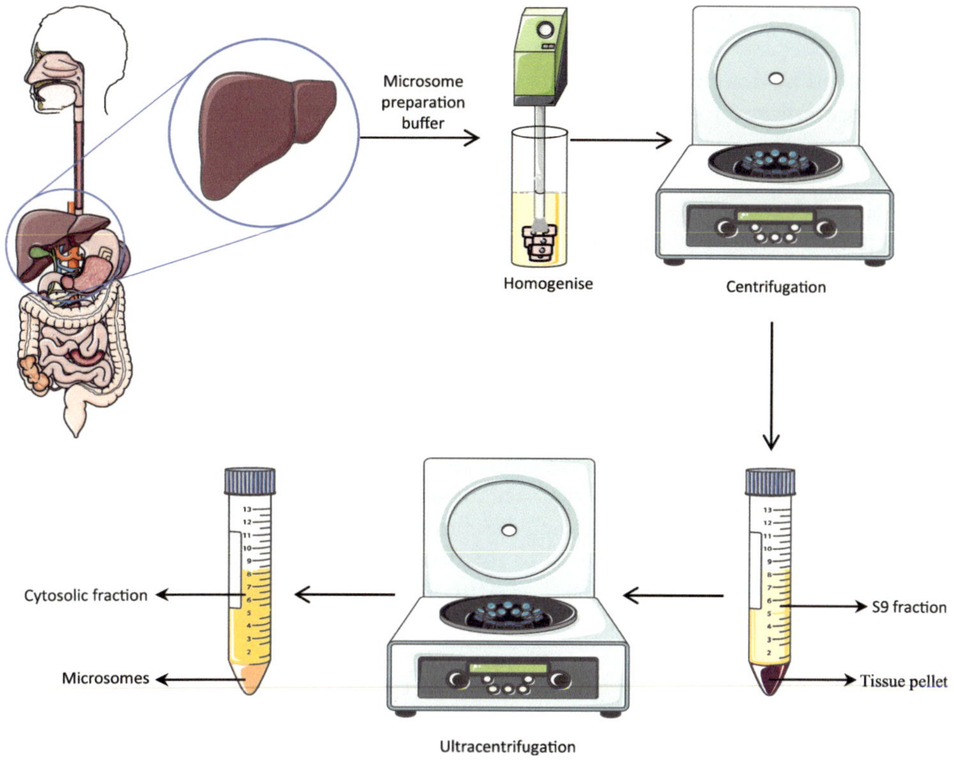

Figure 2.
Preparation of human liver microsomes. Microsome preparation buffer composition: 10 mM potassium phosphate buffer, pH 7.4, with 1.15% (w/v) potassium chloride. Homogenize the liver twice at 20,500 rpm, each time for 30 s, with a 30 s cooling period between bursts. Centrifuge the homogenate for 5 min at 1000 × g, 4°C, then increase to 10,000 × g for a further 10 min. Ultracentrifuge the S9 fraction for 60 min at 105,000 × g, 4°C.

prerequisites [5, 8, 37]. HLM are preferred as they are simple, economical, easy to store for long-term usage, and offer high throughput screening. Nevertheless, HLM has few drawbacks as it is unsuitable for quantitative assessments in drug metabolism studies since it lacks *N*-acetyltransferase (NAT), glutathione-S-transferase (GST), sulfotransferase (SULT) enzymes, and other cofactors. This drawback restricts the competitiveness in metabolism as well as limits the generation of a few metabolites. It also fails to consider the percentage of drugs bound to plasma proteins instead of microsomes crucial for *in vivo* metabolism studies [5, 8, 36, 37].

4. Drug metabolism studies by HLM

CYP activity changes in different species and this interspecies variation in drug metabolism can be estimated by investigating the *in vitro* drug metabolism in liver microsomes obtained from various species. The appropriate animal model for pharmacokinetics and toxicological studies can be determined by comparing the CYP metabolic profiles obtained from different species with the HLM. Microsomes can be acquired from the below-stated corporations: XenoTech LLC (www.xenotechllc.com), Human Biologics (www.humanbiologics.com), Cedra, Co. (www.cedracorp.com), BD Gentest (www.bdbiosciences.com) and Celsis International (www.celsis.com).

However, it is to be noted that the activity of the microsomes fluctuates among different batches and vendors. For instance, rat liver microsomes obtained from two different vendors demonstrated significant activity differences in the biotransformation of buspirone and loperamide. In contrast, the one obtained from the third vendor showed no activity. Furthermore, three batches obtained from the same supplier exhibited different activities in the biotransformation of buspirone and loperamide [39]. These differences were observed because of the innate differences in animals and varying preparation methods chosen by the vendors. Few vendors prepare liver microsomes by using phenylmethylsulfonylfluoride, while others use ethylenediaminetetraacetic acid (EDTA). Phenylmethylsulfonylfluoride inhibits trypsin-like proteases that are responsible for microsomal proteolytic degradation and certain carboxylesterases. On the other hand, EDTA chelates calcium and iron inhibiting both calcium-dependent phospholipases and lipid peroxidation. For each fresh batch, it is vital to examine the microsomal characterization data given by the vendor to check the CYP content, cytochrome b5, and NADPH-cytochrome c reductase activity.

For quantifying metabolites, drugs are incubated with microsomes with a low microsomal protein concentration, i.e., ≤0.5 mg/mL [40, 41]. This low concentration reduces the extent of protein binding to the drug. The final protein concentration of preparation is assessed by a Bradford protein assay or Lowry protein assay with bovine serum albumin as a standard. Storage of HLM at low temperatures (−80°C) maintains the activity of CYP enzymes for an extended period [40]. Microsomes thawed and kept on ice for less than 2 hours can be re-frozen at −80°C for reuse as there will be insignificant loss of enzyme activity [42].

The drug concentration used *in vitro* studies is higher than that observed in blood in an animal study. When the *in vivo* drug concentrations are unknown, the final drug concentration is chosen from a range of 1–10 μM to simulate the *in vivo* conditions. Drug's incubating concentrations (0.5–15 μM) have a significant influence on the drug's stability consequences: higher concentrations of the drug are more stable in microsomes [39]. Thus, it is recommended to work with two different concentrations of a drug for understanding the concentration impact on its stability within the microsomes and additional matrices. Low concentrations of the drug are proposed for *in vitro* studies due to the following reasons: 1) The reaction between the test drug and enzyme follows a first-order reaction, i.e., the rate of the reaction is directly proportional to the concentration of the drug 2) Concentration of organic solvents always should be low as it reduces the microsomal activity.

The control groups should exclude the substrate, microsomes, NADPH, or the NRS from the incubation solution. Ice-cold organic solvent (e.g., acetonitrile or methanol) is used to quench the reaction. Incubation time of less than 2 h at 37°C is suggested for performing a stability study using microsomes [42]. In the extended incubation period, additional control group incubations need to be included to ensure the enzyme's activity and thermal degradation of the drug. When metabolite identification is difficult, the % of unchanged parent drug versus time will be recorded. Organic solvents employed for solubilizing lipophilic drugs inhibit CYP activity. DMSO concentrations of 0.2, 0.5, or 1% inhibit the CYP activity resulting in erroneous stability data of incubated drugs. DMSO specifically inhibits CYP2E1, and hence, it should be avoided for studies involving the CYP2E1 enzyme. Organic solvents like methanol, ethanol, acetonitrile, and PEG 400 also inhibit about 15–25% of CYP2E1, CYP3A4, CYP2D6, CYP2C9, and CYP2C19 activity. The permissible limits for the organic solvents in solubilizing the drugs while retaining the CYP activity are methanol <1.0%, acetonitrile <1.0% and DMSO <0.2% [11].

4.1 Reaction phenotyping studies

Reaction phenotyping, also known as enzyme mapping, helps determine the enzymes involved in the metabolism of a specific drug. The data from these studies are essential in identifying potential drug interactions with common co-medications. Further, these studies help in anticipating possible pharmacokinetic changes caused by genetic polymorphisms in certain enzymes. Understanding the role of a specific enzyme involved in the metabolism of a drug is vital in the following conditions: 1) Identifying potential DDI with concomitant medications that may be inhibitors or inducers of the same enzymes [43]. 2) Establishing the metabolism of a drug by an enzyme that exhibits genetic polymorphism may result in significant inter-individual variability [44]. 3) Determining the formation of pharmacologically active metabolites [45]. 4) Deducing the extent of drug metabolism and the generation of significant metabolites [45].

In general, *in vitro* reaction phenotyping studies helps identify and characterize the formation of significant metabolites in drug metabolism at the preclinical stage. Toxicological studies assess the safety of these metabolites. In addition to toxicological considerations, detecting any pharmacological effects of major metabolites is also essential. Human radiolabel mass balance studies before phase III trials unravel main elimination pathways and systemic metabolite exposure. Data from the human radiolabel mass balance and the *in vitro* studies confirm metabolic pathways and the enzymes responsible for the drug metabolism. The CYP and non-CYP enzymes that contribute to ≥25% of drug elimination should be uncovered. The *in vivo* contribution is assessed by interaction with a potent, selective inhibitor or pharmacogenetic studies to decipher elimination pathways [46]. Assessment of reaction phenotyping uses approaches such as recombinantly expressed enzymes and correlation analysis. Recombinantly expressed enzymes use scaling methods like the relative activity factor (RAF) or the intersystem extrapolation factor (ISEF) for interpreting the relative contribution of the individual enzymes. The correlation analysis utilizes pooled HLM obtained from at least 10 donors for testing the activity toward respective probe substrates [47].

4.2 Enzyme inhibition studies

Enzyme inhibition experiments evaluate known CYP enzyme inhibitors on the metabolism of a drug by either pooled HLM or individual CYP isoforms. The usage of selective chemical inhibitors allows easy illustration of the metabolic pathways. To prevent false results, careful estimation of the drug and inhibitor concentrations for incubation is a must. Higher inhibitor concentrations exhibit non-selective chemical inhibition. For instance, quinidine and ketoconazole at <1 μM concentration act as selective CYP2D6 and CYP3A4 inhibitors. Although, at higher concentrations, these drugs inhibit other CYP isoforms as well. Chemical CYP inhibition is categorized into two types: reversible (could be competitive inhibition or non-competitive inhibition) and irreversible inhibition. In irreversible inhibition ("mechanism-based inhibition" or "suicide inhibition"), the CYP enzyme metabolizes the drug into a reactive metabolite that firmly binds to the enzyme's active site leading to a prolonged inactivation [48, 49]. These studies can be conducted before or after carrying out the cDNA-expressed recombinant CYP enzyme studies. They impart extra proof to assist the cDNA-expressed recombinant CYPs study results. Further, they may also provide a direction to these studies for the active isoform identification.

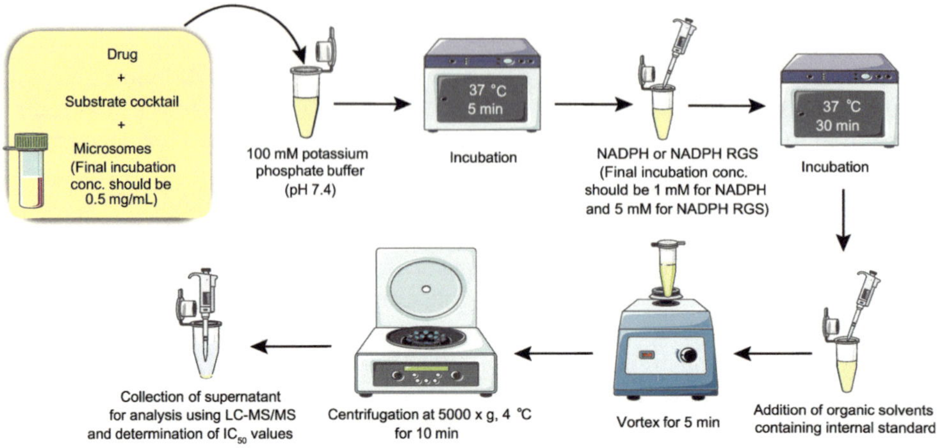

Figure 3.
Workflow to assess enzyme inhibition using human liver microsomes.

Figure 3 demonstrates the protocol for the CYP inhibition study. The procedure involves incubating the drug with liver microsomes in the presence and absence of selective inhibitors at 37°C for 30 min [40]. The following inhibitors against the isoforms and their concentrations are recommended: furafylline (CYP1A2; 0.1, 1, 10 μM), 8- glitazones or quercetin (CYP2C8; 0.5, 1, 10 μM), quinidine (CYP2D6, 0.5, 1, 10 μM), sulphaphenazole (CYP2C19; 5, 20, 100 μM), methoxypsoralen (CYP2A6; 0.1, 1, 10 μM), troleandomycin (TAO; CYP3A, 0.5, 1, 10 μM), clomethiazole (CYP2E1, 0.1,1,10 μM) [40, 50]. Methanol (< 1% (v/v) of the entire mixture) is used to dissolve the inhibitors before adding them to the incubation mixture. Prior to drug addition, inhibitors undergo preincubation at 37°C, with NADPH and microsomes, reaching a final concentration of 10 mM. A positive control is carried out in the presence of the drug with 1% methanol in the incubation mixture, whereas a blank control lacks the drug. Thus, the control values are employed to successfully determine the percentage of inhibition observed in the metabolite generation.

Conventionally, *in vitro* CYP enzyme inhibition studies were conducted using HLM, for which isoform-specific substrates were incubated along with the investigational drug. At the end of the incubation, the formation of the metabolite is monitored by analytical techniques like high-performance liquid chromatography (HPLC), liquid chromatography coupled with mass spectrometry (LC-/MS), or fluorescence and this procedure is repeated for at least three different concentrations of that drug [51, 52]. Identification of many drug molecules in the drug discovery process is possible using combinatorial chemistry approaches and high throughput screening techniques.

4.3 Drug metabolite profiling

Metabolite profiling refers to the relative quantification, identification, and characterization of the number of metabolites formed in the biological matrices. These studies help researchers structurally and chemically modify the drug to increase its efficacy, reduce its toxicity, and facilitate the synthesis of a molecule with enhanced therapeutic activity [53–56]. The FDA guidance "Safety Testing of Drug Metabolites" states that the metabolic drug profile must be determined by *in vitro* and *in vivo* models at various phases of the drug development. *In vitro* metabolite profiling of a drug can be performed using liver microsomes, hepatocytes or liver slices collected from humans or animals [57]. The regulatory bodies (ICH, EMEA, and FDA) recommend studying *in-vitro* and *in-vivo* hepatic drug metabolismFDA guidance mentions the importance of metabolism studies via the kidney and the gastrointestinal tract as most orally administered medications interact with the gastrointestinal enzymes [58, 59]. Other regulatory authorities lay minimal emphasis on extra-hepatic metabolism studies.

Using a single high concentration of drug or a series of concentrations produces a high concentration of metabolites that meets the demands of quantification. A concentration of 50 μM or concentrations of 5, 50, and 500 μM can be chosen for novel metabolites. Concentration should be higher than or equal to the K_m value (Michaelis constant) recorded for the CYP substrates to generate metabolites in measurable amounts. A positive control having testosterone or phenacetin should be included for measuring the formation of 6β-hydroxytestosterone acetaminophen metabolites. A negative control without NADPH for each test compound helps determine the sources of metabolites other than oxidative metabolism (e.g., carboxylesterases, nonenzymatic metabolite formation, substrate impurities) [11].

4.4 Metabolic stability

Metabolic stability defines the liability of a drug compound to its metabolism. It is determined by estimating the disappearance of the drug substrate in a relevant *in vitro* system over a particular period. Further, metabolic stability data gives information on the secondary pharmacokinetic parameters such as bioavailability and half-life of the drug. Therefore, optimizing metabolic stability plays a vital role in the drug discovery and development phase [60]. These obtained parameters explain the drug's pharmacological and toxicological profile and shed light on the patient adherence to the drug. **Figure 4** shows the different stages in the metabolic stability study.

Metabolic stability studies are performed at a drug concentration less than K_m value, where enzymatic reactions follow the first-order process. While dealing with an unknown K_m value, 1 μM concentration of a drug is recommended. In general, the metabolic system is incubated with the drug substrate for a specified period at 37°C. The disappearance of the drug substrate is monitored at individual time points using a

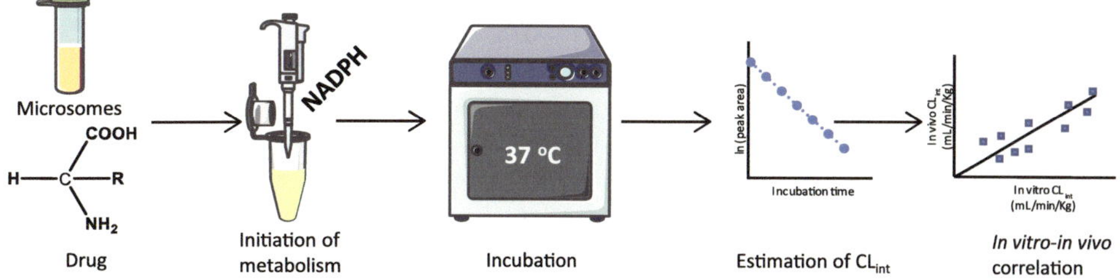

Figure 4.
Metabolic stability of drug substance. This assessment involves the incubation of the drug with microsomes in 100 mM potassium phosphate buffer. The addition of 1 mM NADPH solution followed by incubation at 37°C initiates the metabolic reaction. The disappearance of the drug substrate is monitored at individual time points using the analytical technique. Plotting the natural log of peak area ratio with time yields a straight line, where the slope of the line gives the elimination rate constant that helps in predicting the intrinsic clearance. The conversion scaling factors involves in the correlation between the clearance values obtained from the in vitro *intrinsic clearance data and* in vivo *clearance values.*

suitable analytical technique. Testosterone or DL-propranolol is added as a positive control to ensure the adequate execution of the assay. A negative control without NADPH is included to ascertain drug loss due to thermal degradation. Negative controls could also serve as matrix controls if they lack the drug or responsible enzyme. Plotting natural log of peak area ratio (drug substance peak area/internal standard peak area) with time yields a straight line, where the slope of the line gives the elimination rate constant (k).

The following equation determines half-life ($t_{1/2}$)

$$t_{\frac{1}{2}} = \frac{0.693}{k}$$

Metabolic stability studies derive various parameters that include half-life, intrinsic clearance, and total hepatic clearance. These parameters can be calculated using "well-stirred" and "parallel tube" approaches. In the "well-stirred" approach, the liver is characterized by a single compartment where the intracellular free concentration of drugs in hepatocytes is in equilibrium with the free concentration of drug in blood eliminating from the liver. Whereas in a "parallel tube" approach, the liver comprises numerous parallel tubes, in which the enzymes are evenly distributed. In every tube, the intracellular free concentration of drug in hepatocytes is in equilibrium with the free concentration of the drug in blood [61].

The whole liver CL_{int} is determined by using *in vitro* half-life:

$$\text{Whole liver } CL_{int} = \frac{0.693 \times \text{liver weight}}{invitrot_{\frac{1}{2}} \times \text{amount of the liver in incubation} \times \text{fraction unbound to microsomal protein}}$$

According to the "well-stirred" model, hepatic clearance (CL_H) and hepatic extraction ratio (E_H) are given by: [62].

$$CL_H = \frac{Q_H \times CL_{int}}{Q_H + CL_{int}}$$

$$E_H = \frac{CL_H}{Q_H}$$

where Q_H is the hepatic blood flow.

4.5 Enzyme kinetics in drug metabolism using HLM

It is essential to determine the enzymes involved in the metabolism process and their respective kinetic parameters throughout the drug discovery process. Enzyme kinetics involves studying reaction rates affected by different experimental variables such as enzyme concentration, substrate concentration, enzyme activators, enzyme inhibitors, temperature, pH, and ionic strength [63, 64]. Chakraborty et al. demonstrated the effect of pH, temperature, pressure and dwell time on enzyme inhibition kinetics in pineapple puree and concluded that the temperature had the highest impact on enzyme inactivation [65]. Further, they elucidate the role of polymorphism in determining drug clearance and aid in predicting drug–drug interactions associated with metabolites [66].

The CYP enzyme family metabolizes numerous xenobiotics, thus making it an integral part of drug–drug interactions [67]. Inhibition studies predict most P450 oxidations and drug–drug interactions, owing to their competitive Michaelis–Menten kinetics. Models with a single binding site are explained by competitive, noncompetitive, and uncompetitive inhibition, or activation of the enzyme, whereas some CYP3A4 oxidations tend to demonstrate unusual kinetics [67, 68]. Michaelis–Menten kinetics determines the enzyme kinetic constants such as K_m and V_{max}. The reaction velocity (V), i.e., the formation rates of metabolites with a fixed amount of HLM, is given by: [69].

$$V = \frac{V_{max} \cdot C}{K_m + C}$$

where C depicts the initial drug concentration, V_{max} gives the maximum reaction velocity of the enzyme, and K_m represents the Michaelis–Menten constant.

Intrinsic clearance (CL_{int}) is defined as the ratio of the rate of product formation to the substrate concentration and can be ascertained by using the K_m and V_{max} values [70].

$$CL_{int} = \frac{\upsilon}{[S]} = \frac{V_{max}}{K_m + [S]}$$

where [S] is the substrate concentration, V_{max} gives the maximum reaction velocity of the enzyme,

and K_m represents the Michaelis–Menten constant.

When the concentration of the substrate is considerably lower than the K_m value, then intrinsic clearance is augmented to total clearance [70]. Then, the above equation is simplified to:

$$CL_{int} \approx \frac{V_{max}}{K_m}$$

In cases where more than one CYP is involved in a drug metabolism reaction, a biphasic relationship is observed between V_{max} (maximal reaction velocity) and [S] (substrate concentration). It can be explained by using a two-enzyme model [8]:

$$V = \frac{V_{max1} \cdot [S]}{K_{m1} + [S]} + \frac{V_{max2} \cdot [S]}{K_{m2} + [S]}$$

Where K_{m1} and K_{m2} are high-affinity and low-affinity component constants, V_{max1} and V_{max2} are the maximal velocities of the enzymes for high and low-affinity components, respectively.

Atypical kinetics are elucidated through a particular enzyme by binding more than one drug molecule concomitantly or through other active site interactions [71, 72]. Hence, it is essential to analyze kinetics as an *in vivo* or *in vitro* effect to prevent an erroneous prediction of intrinsic clearance and ultimately impact the *in vivo* clearance [72]. Eadie-Hofstee plots are used to resolve multiple-enzyme kinetics when Michaelis–Menten plots fail to be beneficial [73]. It is essential to model the non-additive interactions to understand multidrug cocktails usage [74]. Further, it is necessary to consider the non-specific binding in enzyme kinetics. The chances of these events are high, resulting in the *in vitro* clearance values being closer to the measured values. However, if the non-specific binding is absent, the obtained values of intrinsic clearance will be lower than the real-time *in vivo* clearance [75].

Electrochemical methods determine enzyme kinetics where electron transfers are involved. The catalytic activity of the cytochrome P450 enzyme is electro analyzed as the catalytic cycle requires electron transfer. Electroanalysis paves the way for multicomponent studies entailing many drugs to describe interactions under the mutual influence or drug interference, which in turn is manifested by an alteration in the kinetic constants of enzymatic catalysis [76]. Novel microfluidic tools and detection methods have made the high throughput measurement of enzyme kinetics possible using droplet-based optofluidic systems [77]. A nanochannel-array enzyme reactor has been developed to comprehend the basics of enzymatic reactions restricted to nano-spaces and also gives an outreach to design productive enzyme reactors [78].

Many *in vitro* systems like HLM, human hepatocytes, recombinantly expressed CYP enzymes, S9 fractions and human liver slices are used to determine the intrinsic clearance of the drug for speculating the *in vivo* clearance by estimating the kinetic parameters, K_m and V_{max} values. HLM is a well-established in vitro system for studying drug metabolism through CYP450 kinetics due to its low cost, ease of use, and commercial availability [79]. CYP activity levels differ in different microsomal preparations. This variation between different donor's preparations can be used to understand the effects of age, sex, and genotype on CYP-regulated kinetics [22].

4.6 Glutathione conjugation assay

The tripeptide, L-γ-glutamyl-L-cysteinyl-glycine, known as Glutathione (GSH), is a low molecular mass, thiol-reducing compound, synthesized from L-glutamate, L-cysteine, and glycine amino acids [80]. The cysteine sulfhydryl group (-SH) is responsible for reduction and conjugation reactions for eliminating reactive electrophiles and enhancing a lipophilic compound's solubility [81, 82]. GSH is usually found at concentrations between 1 and 10 mM and involves scavenging reactive oxygen species and detoxifying foreign compounds [83, 84]. The glutathione conjugation is followed by a series of metabolic and transport phases that eventually leads to the mercapturic acid formation (S-conjugates of N-acetylcysteine) [85, 86]. The formed mercapturic acid is more polar and, thus, easily excreted in urine [87]. Glutathione S-transferases (GSTs) include drug-metabolizing enzymes responsible for catalyzing glutathione conjugation with many foreign compounds [88]. They belong to the superfamily of Phase II enzymes and exist as dimeric proteins [89, 90].

The human GST is present in the cytosol, is expressed in the liver, and is subdivided into classes α, π, and μ. In a human liver, 80–90% of the GST is present in the form of GST-α [91]. The expression of these GST-α enzymes may lead to resistance toward anticancer drugs, and thus, GSTs can also be used as markers for malignant tumors [92, 93]. The main functions of GSTs are redox signaling, antioxidation, and detoxification of many cancer drugs [94–96]. The detoxification phenomenon is not always valid, and in some instances, GSH S-conjugates were observed to be toxic [97]. Christoph Englert et al. reported that nanocarriers' coupling to glutathione aided in effectively crossing the blood–brain barrier [98].

4.7 Glucuronidation and its kinetics

Glucuronidation reaction results in the conjugation of glucuronic acid obtained from uridine diphosphate-glucuronic acid (UDPGA) to compounds that contain hydroxyl, carboxyl, thiol, amino, and acidic functional groups by UDP-glucuronosyltransferase enzymes (UGTs) [99, 100]. UGTs are abundant in the liver and intestine [101]. These membrane-bound enzymes of the endoplasmic reticulum account for the metabolism of more than 35% of drugs [102, 103]. Human UGT enzymes are categorized into four families, namely: UGT1, UGT2, UGT3, and UGT8. These enzymes are further classified into UGT 1A, 2A, and 2B isoforms depending upon the structure of the gene and the analogy of sequence. The isoforms expressed in the liver of UGT1A: UGT1A1, UGT1A3, UGT1A4, UGT1A5, UGT1A6, and UGT1A9 [104, 105] and UGT2B isoforms: UGT2B4, UGT2B7, UGT2B10, UGT2B11, UGT2B15, UGT2B17 and UGT2B28 [104]. The lumen of the endoplasmic reticulum (ER) serves as an active site for UGTs, and its membrane allows substrates, cofactors, and products to diffuse [106]. The latent action of the UGTs in microsomal incubations can be removed by distorting the barrier. Alamethicin disrupts the barrier by forming pores in the membrane and permits entry to the enzyme, causing no impact on the membrane's structure or its intrinsic catalytic activity [107]. Glucuronidation is a detoxification reaction as it enhances the compound's polarity and facilitates the excretion of compounds through urine and bile [103, 108]. It is necessary to comprehend the involvement of UGTs in the drug's metabolism as it aids in averting drug–drug interactions and adverse drug reactions [109].

In the first stage, the microsomes are activated in 0.1 M potassium phosphate buffer (pH 7.4) pre-incubated with 50 μg/mL concentration of alamethicin on ice for 30 min. The drug is incubated for 5 min at 37°C with 0.1 M potassium phosphate buffer (pH 7.4), 4 mM $MgCl_2$and the activated HLM with the final concentration of 0.5 mg/mL. The metabolic reaction is initiated by adding 5 mM UDPGA and incubating this mixture at 37°C for predetermined time points. A well-known UGT substrate is included as a positive control, and a mixture without UDPGA is used as a negative control to assess the formation of metabolites other than glucuronidation metabolism [110, 111]. The addition of ice-cold extraction solvents (Acetonitrile or methanol) terminates the reaction. The samples are centrifuged, and the supernatant is collected for further analysis using a suitable analytical technique like HPLC [112–114] or LC–MS/MS [115–117].

Kinetic analyses were performed with HLM and commercially available UGTs. The elucidation of the kinetics of glucuronidation has a significant influence on the credibility of the predicted *in vitro* clearance value [118]. Michaelis–Menten kinetic model is used for the determination of the kinetics of glucuronidation via kinetic constants, K_m (Michaelis constant, the concentration of substrate when the reaction rate is 50% of V_{max}) and V_{max} (the maximum rate of reaction when the substrate saturates all the active sites of the enzymes). Kinetics of glucuronidation for several drugs like NSAIDs [119], olanzapine [120], serotonin [121], and ursolic acid [122] were determined using this model. The substrate inhibition equation used is:

$$\nu = \frac{V_{max}\,[S]}{K_s + [S] + {}^{[S]^2}/_{K_{si}}}$$

where v is the reaction rate, [S] is the substrate concentration, V_{max} is the maximum velocity, K_s is the substrate affinity constant, and K_{si} is the substrate inhibition constant [123].

The hill equation is used to determine the sigmoidal kinetics:

$$\nu = \frac{V_{max}\,S^n}{S_{50}^n + S^n}$$

where S_{50}^{n} is the substrate concentration leading to 50% of V_{max}, and n is the Hill coefficient [124].

Eadie–Hofstee plots and Lineweaver-Burk plots determine the model to be selected for the kinetic analyses using nonlinear regression analysis for fitting the experimental data [125, 126]. A straight line in the plot signifies the Michaelis–Menten model's usage. In contrast, if a hook in the upper panel is obtained, it represents the usage of the substrate inhibition model [110, 127].

5. Conclusion

After the drug's oral administration, the drug undergoes various processes like absorption, distribution, metabolism, and excretion. Metabolism of most of the drugs is carried out by CYP and UGT enzymes, which are abundant in the liver. *In vivo* and *in vitro* studies are often used for drug metabolism studies. *In vivo* studies involve screening serum, urine and feces, whereas *in vitro* drug metabolism studies are carried out using HLM, human hepatocytes, and recombinantly expressed cytochrome P450 enzymes. HLM are widely used as it offers several advantages like high throughput screening, ease in storage, economic, and simplicity and convenience in their usage. Metabolism studies play a significant role in identifying, characterizing, and quantifying potential metabolites of a particular drug, thereby elucidating the drug metabolism pathway. Metabolism may convert a drug into a toxic metabolite or render an inactive drug into its active form. Metabolic stability helps predict the metabolic clearance of the drug and thereby helps in dosage adjustment and the frequency of administration of a drug. Therefore, conducting drug metabolism studies using HLM at the drug discovery stage helps screen the potential leads with optimized pharmacological properties.

Acknowledgements

The authors are grateful to the Department of Pharmaceuticals, Ministry of Chemicals & Fertilizers, Government of India, New Delhi, for the award of the NIPER fellowship. The manuscript bears the NIPER-Hyderabad communication number NIPER-H/2021/210.

Conflict of interest

The authors declare no conflict of interest.

Author details

Siva Nageswara Rao Gajula, Sakina Asgar Vora, Amol G. Dikundwar and Rajesh Sonti*
Department of Pharmaceutical Analysis, National Institute of Pharmaceutical Education and Research (NIPER), Hyderabad, Balanagar, Telangana, India

*Address all correspondence to: rajesh.sonti@niperhyd.ac.in; raj.sonti@gmail.com

References

[1] Koster A et al. Introduction to Pharmacogenesis. Utrecht, The Netherlands: Faculty of Pharmaceutical Sciences; 1997

[2] Burns J. Fundamental of Drug Metabolism and Drug Disposition. In: BN La Du, HG Mandel and EL Way, The Williams and Wilkins Co., Baltimore, 1972: p. 352-353

[3] Gaunitz F et al. In vitro metabolic profiling of synthetic cannabinoids by pooled human liver microsomes, cytochrome P450 isoenzymes, and Cunninghamella elegans and their detection in urine samples. Analytical and Bioanalytical Chemistry. 2019; **411**(16):3561-3579

[4] Rane A, Wilkinson G, Shand D. Prediction of hepatic extraction ratio from in vitro measurement of intrinsic clearance. Journal of Pharmacology and Experimental Therapeutics. 1977;**200**(2): 420-424

[5] Fasinu P, Bouic PJ, Rosenkranz B. Liver-based in vitro technologies for drug biotransformation studies-a review. Current Drug Metabolism. 2012;**13**(2): 215-224

[6] Dalvie D et al. Assessment of three human in vitro systems in the generation of major human excretory and circulating metabolites. Chemical Research in Toxicology. 2009;**22**(2): 357-368

[7] Gunaratna C. Drug metabolism & pharmacokinetics in drug discovery: A primer for bioanalytical chemists, part I. Current Separations. 2000;**19**(1):17-24

[8] Asha S, Vidyavathi M. Role of human liver microsomes in in vitro metabolism of drugs—A review. Applied Biochemistry and Biotechnology. 2010; **160**(6):1699-1722

[9] Castro-Perez JM. Current and future trends in the application of HPLC-MS to metabolite-identification studies. Drug Discovery Today. 2007;**12**(5–6):249-256

[10] Guengerich FP et al. Introduction: Drug metabolism and toxicology special issue. Journal of Medicinal Chemistry. ACS Publications; 2020;**63**:6249-6250

[11] Knights KM et al. In vitro drug metabolism using liver microsomes. Current Protocols in Pharmacology. 2016;**74**(1):7.8. 1-7.8. 24

[12] Coleman MD. Human Drug Metabolism. Boschstr., Weinheim, Germany: John Wiley & Sons; 2019

[13] Li Y et al. Current trends in drug metabolism and pharmacokinetics. Acta Pharmaceutica Sinica B. 2019;**9**(6): 1113-1144

[14] Hu B et al. Structure–property relationships and machine learning models for addressing CYP3A4-mediated victim drug–drug interaction risk in drug discovery. Molecular Pharmaceutics. 2020;**17**(9):3600-3608

[15] Sheweita SA. Drug-metabolizing enzymes mechanisms and functions. Current Drug Metabolism. 2000;**1**(2): 107-132

[16] Caldwell J, Gardner I, Swales N. An Introduction to Drug Disposition: The Basic Principles of Absorption, Distribution, Metabolism, and Excretion. Thousand Oaks, CA: Sage Publications Sage CA; 1995

[17] Jaladanki CK et al. Mechanistic studies on the drug metabolism and

toxicity originating from cytochromes P450. Drug Metabolism Reviews. 2020; **52**:1-29

[18] Caira MR, Ionescu C. Drug Metabolism: Current Concepts. Vol. 7. Dordrecht, Netherlands: Springer Science & Business Media; 2006

[19] Testa B, Kraemer SD. The biochemistry of drug metabolism–an introduction: Part 5. Metabolism and bioactivity. Chemistry & Biodiversity. 2009;**6**(5):591-684

[20] Midha KK, Rawson MJ, Hubbard JW. The role of metabolites in bioequivalence. Pharmaceutical Research. 2004;**21**(8):1331-1344

[21] Russell LE et al. Advances in the study of drug metabolism–symposium report of the 12th meeting of the International Society for the Study of xenobiotics (ISSX). Drug Metabolism Reviews. 2020;**52**:1-13

[22] Krämer SD, Testa B. The biochemistry of drug metabolism–an introduction: Part 6. Inter-individual factors affecting drug metabolism. Chemistry & Biodiversity. 2008;**5**(12): 2465-2578

[23] Kraemer SD, Testa B. The biochemistry of drug metabolism–an introduction: Part 7. Intra-individual factors affecting drug metabolism. Chemistry & Biodiversity. 2009;**6**(10): 1477-1660

[24] Gibson GG, Skett P. Factors affecting drug metabolism: Internal factors. In: Introduction to Drug Metabolism. Boston MA: Springer; 1986. pp. 113-146

[25] Mucklow J. Environmental factors affecting drug metabolism. Pharmacology & Therapeutics. 1988; **36**(1):105-117

[26] Durnas C, Loi C-M, Cusack BJ. Hepatic drug metabolism and aging. Clinical Pharmacokinetics. 1990;**19**(5): 359-389

[27] Lammers LA et al. The effects of fasting on drug metabolism. Expert Opinion on Drug Metabolism & Toxicology. 2020;**16**(1):79-85

[28] Camenisch G, Umehara KI. Predicting human hepatic clearance from in vitro drug metabolism and transport data: A scientific and pharmaceutical perspective for assessing drug–drug interactions. Biopharmaceutics & Drug Disposition. 2012;**33**(4): 179-194

[29] Riley RJ, Grime K. Metabolic screening in vitro: Metabolic stability, CYP inhibition and induction. Drug Discovery Today: Technologies. 2004; **1**(4):365-372

[30] Ekins S et al. Present and future in vitro approaches for drug metabolism. Journal of Pharmacological and Toxicological Methods. 2000;**44**(1): 313-324

[31] Horspool AM et al. Human liver Microsomes immobilized on Magnetizable beads: A novel approach to study In vitro drug metabolism. Drug Metabolism and Disposition. 2020; **48**(8):645-654

[32] Wrighton SA et al. In vitro methods for assessing human hepatic drug metabolism: Their use in drug development. Drug Metabolism Reviews. 1993;**25**(4):453-484

[33] Ball S et al. The application of in vitro models of drug metabolism and

toxicity in drug discovery and drug development. Drug and Chemical Toxicology. 1995;**18**(1):1-28

[34] Eliesen GA et al. Toxicity of anticancer drugs in human placental tissue explants and trophoblast cell lines. Archives of Toxicology. 2020;**95**: 1-15

[35] Lušin TT, Trontelj J, Mrhar A. Raloxifene glucuronidation in human intestine, kidney, and liver microsomes and in human liver microsomes genotyped for the UGT1A1* 28 polymorphism. Drug Metabolism and Disposition. 2011;**39**(12):2347-2354

[36] Hariparsad N et al. In vitro methods in human drug biotransformation research: Implications for cancer chemotherapy. Toxicology In Vitro. 2006;**20**(2):135-153

[37] Brandon EF et al. An update on in vitro test methods in human hepatic drug biotransformation research: Pros and cons. Toxicology and Applied Pharmacology. 2003;**189**(3):233-246

[38] Jia L, Liu X. The conduct of drug metabolism studies considered good practice (II): in vitro experiments. Current Drug Metabolism. 2007;**8**(8): 822-829

[39] Di L et al. Optimization of a higher throughput microsomal stability screening assay for profiling drug discovery candidates. Journal of Biomolecular Screening. 2003;**8**(4): 453-462

[40] Bjornsson TD et al. The conduct of in vitro and in vivo drug-drug interaction studies: A pharmaceutical research and manufacturers of America (PhRMA) perspective. Drug Metabolism and Disposition. 2003;**31**(7):815-832

[41] Projean D et al. In vitro metabolism of chloroquine: Identification of CYP2C8, CYP3A4, and CYP2D6 as the main isoforms catalyzing N-desethyl chloroquine formation. Drug Metabolism and Disposition. 2003;**31**(6):748-754

[42] Pearce RE et al. Effects of freezing, thawing, and storing human liver microsomes on cytochrome P450 activity. Archives of Biochemistry and Biophysics. 1996;**331**(2):145-169

[43] Ogilvie BW et al. In vitro approaches for studying the inhibition of drug-metabolizing enzymes and identifying the drug-metabolizing enzymes responsible for the metabolism of drugs (reaction phenotyping) with emphasis on cytochrome P450. In: Drug-Drug Interactions. Boca Raton: CRC Press; 2008. pp. 231-358

[44] Zhang H et al. Cytochrome P450 reaction-phenotyping: An industrial perspective. Expert Opinion on Drug Metabolism & Toxicology. 2007;**3**(5): 667-687

[45] Chen Y, Mao J, Fretland AJ. Reaction phenotyping. Encyclopedia of Drug Metabolism and Interactions. Hoboken, NJ: John Wiley & Sons; 2011. pp. 1-26

[46] Agency EM. Guideline on the Investigation of Drug Interactions. United Kingdom: European Medicines Agency London; 2012

[47] Chen Y et al. Utility of intersystem extrapolation factors in early reaction phenotyping and the quantitative extrapolation of human liver microsomal intrinsic clearance using recombinant cytochromes P450. Drug Metabolism and Disposition. 2011;**39**(3):373-382

[48] Fontana E, Dansette P, Poli S. Cytochrome p450 enzymes mechanism based inhibitors: Common sub-

structures and reactivity. Current Drug Metabolism. 2005;**6**(5):413-451

[49] Rao Gajula SN et al. Pharmacokinetic drug–drug interactions: An insight into recent US FDA-approved drugs for prostate cancer. Bioanalysis. 2020;**12**(22):1647-1664

[50] Salva M et al. Identification of the human liver enzymes involved in the metabolism of the antimigraine agent almotriptan. Drug Metabolism and Disposition. 2003;**31**(4):404-411

[51] Li G et al. High-throughput cytochrome P450 cocktail inhibition assay for assessing drug-drug and drug-botanical interactions. Drug Metabolism and Disposition. 2015;**43**(11):1670-1678

[52] Fowler S, Zhang H. In vitro evaluation of reversible and irreversible cytochrome P450 inhibition: Current status on methodologies and their utility for predicting drug–drug interactions. The AAPS Journal. 2008;**10**(2):410-424

[53] Wu W, McKown L. Recent advances in biotransformation of CNS and cardiovascular agents. Current Drug Metabolism. 2000;**1**(3):255-270

[54] Uetrecht J. Is it possible to more accurately predict which drug candidates will cause idiosyncratic drug reactions. Current Drug Metabolism. 2000;**1**(2):133-141

[55] White RE. High-throughput screening in drug metabolism and pharmacokinetic support of drug discovery. Annual Review of Pharmacology and Toxicology. 2000;**40**(1):133-157

[56] Li AP. Screening for human ADME/Tox drug properties in drug discovery. Drug Discovery Today. 2001;**6**(7):357-366

[57] Food U. Drug administration guidance for industry, drug metabolism/drug interaction studies in the drug development process: Studies in vitro. Center for Drug Evaluation and Research. 1997

[58] Guideline IHT. Guidance on non-clinical safety studies for the conduct of human clinical trials and marketing authorization for pharmaceuticals M3 (R2). In: International Conference on Harmonisation of Technical Requirements for Registration of Pharmaceuticals for Human Use. 2009

[59] Baillie TA et al. Drug metabolites in safety testing. Toxicology and Applied Pharmacology. 2002;**182**(3):188-196

[60] Gajula SNR, Nadimpalli N, Sonti R. Drug metabolic stability in early drug discovery to develop potential Lead compounds. Drug Metabolism Reviews, 2021;**53**:1-47

[61] Baranczewski P et al. Introduction to in vitro estimation of metabolic stability and drug interactions of new chemical entities in drug discovery and development. Pharmacological Reports. 2006;**58**(4):453

[62] Watanabe S, Kuzhiumparambil U, Fu S. In vitro metabolism of synthetic cannabinoid AM1220 by human liver microsomes and Cunninghamella elegans using liquid chromatography coupled with high resolution mass spectrometry. Forensic Toxicology. 2018;**36**(2):435-446

[63] Lennarz WJ, Lane MD. Encyclopedia of Biological Chemistry. London, UK: Academic Press; 2013

[64] Roskoski R. Michaelis-Menten kinetics. In: Reference Module in

Biomedical Science. Amsterdam, Netherlands: Elservier; 2015

[65] Chakraborty S, Rao PS, Mishra H. Effect of pH on enzyme inactivation kinetics in high-pressure processed pineapple (Ananas comosus L.) puree using response surface methodology. Food and Bioprocess Technology. 2014; **7**(12):3629-3645

[66] Baranczewski P, Edlund PO, Postlind H. Characterization of the cytochrome P450 enzymes and enzyme kinetic parameters for metabolism of BVT. 2938 using different in vitro systems. Journal of Pharmaceutical and Biomedical Analysis. 2006;**40**(5):1121-1130

[67] Korzekwa KR. In vitro enzyme kinetics applied to drug-metabolizing enzymes. Drug-Drug Interactions. 2002; **116**:33-54

[68] Shou M et al. Enzyme kinetics of cytochrome P450-mediated reactions. Current Drug Metabolism. 2001;**2**(1): 17-36

[69] Berk Z. Food Process Engineering and Technology. London, UK: Academic Press; 2018

[70] Seibert E, Tracy TS. Fundamentals of enzyme kinetics. In: Enzyme Kinetics in Drug Metabolism. Totowa, NJ: Springer; 2014. pp. 9-22

[71] Leow JWH, Chan ECY. Atypical Michaelis-Menten kinetics in cytochrome P450 enzymes: A focus on substrate inhibition. Biochemical Pharmacology. 2019;**169**:113615

[72] Christensen H et al. Different enzyme kinetics of midazolam in recombinant CYP3A4 microsomes from human and insect sources. Drug Metabolism and Pharmacokinetics. 2009;**24**(3):261-268

[73] Tweedie DJ. Case study 7. Compiled Aha moments in enzyme kinetics: Authors. In: Experiences, in Enzyme Kinetics in Drug Metabolism. Totowa, NJ: Springer; 2014. pp. 513-519

[74] Finn NA, Kemp ML. Systems biology approaches to enzyme kinetics: Analyzing network models of drug metabolism. In: Enzyme Kinetics in Drug Metabolism. Totowa, NJ: Springer; 2014. pp. 317-334

[75] Waters NJ, Obach RS, Di L. Consideration of the unbound drug concentration in enzyme kinetics. In: Enzyme Kinetics in Drug Metabolism. Totowa, NJ: Springer; 2014. pp. 119-145

[76] Shumyantseva VV et al. From electrochemistry to enzyme kinetics of cytochrome P450. Biosensors and Bioelectronics. 2018;**121**:192-204

[77] Hess D, Yang T, Stavrakis S. Droplet-based optofluidic systems for measuring enzyme kinetics. Analytical and Bioanalytical Chemistry. 2020;**412**(14): 3265-3283

[78] Li SJ et al. Real-time monitoring of mass-transport-related enzymatic reaction kinetics in a Nanochannel-Array reactor. Chemistry–a. European Journal. 2010;**16**(33):10186-10194

[79] Venkatakrishnan K, von Moltke LL, Greenblatt DJ. Human drug metabolism and the cytochromes P450: Application and relevance of in vitro models. The Journal of Clinical Pharmacology. 2001; **41**(11):1149-1179

[80] Sies H. Glutathione and its role in cellular functions. Free Radical Biology and Medicine. 1999;**27**(9–10):916-921

[81] Forman HJ, Zhang H, Rinna A. Glutathione: Overview of its protective

roles, measurement, and biosynthesis. Molecular Aspects of Medicine. 2009;**30** (1–2):1-12

[82] Hayes J, Wolf C. Role of Glutathione Transferase in Drug Resistance. London, UK: Academic Press; 1988. pp. 3150-3355

[83] Scirè A et al. Glutathione compartmentalization and its role in glutathionylation and other regulatory processes of cellular pathways. BioFactors. 2019;**45**(2): 152-168

[84] Zhong L et al. Formation of glutathione patulin conjugates associated with yeast fermentation contributes to patulin reduction. Food Control. 2020; **123**:107334

[85] Hinchman CA, Ballatori N. Glutathione conjugation and conversion to mercapturic acids can occur as an intrahepatic process. Journal of Toxicology and Environmental Health, Part A Current Issues. 1994;**41**(4): 387-409

[86] Monks TJ, Lau SS. Glutathione conjugation as a mechanism for the transport of reactive metabolites. Advances in Pharmacology. Elsevier; 1994;**27**:183-210

[87] Lash LH. Glutathione-dependent bioactivation. Current Protocols in Toxicology. 2007;**34**(1):6.12. 1-6.12. 16

[88] Chasseaud L. The nature and distribution of enzymes catalyzing the conjugation of glutathione with foreign compounds. Drug Metabolism Reviews. 1974;**2**(1):185-220

[89] Sundberg K et al. Glutathione conjugation and DNA adduct formation of dibenzo [a, l] pyrene and benzo [a] pyrene diol epoxides in V79 cells stably expressing different human glutathione transferases. Chemical Research in Toxicology. 2002;**15**(2):170-179

[90] Van Bladeren PJ. Glutathione conjugation as a bioactivation reaction. Chemico-Biological Interactions. 2000; **129**(1–2):61-76

[91] Gibbs JP, Czerwinski M, Slattery JT. Busulfan-glutathione conjugation catalyzed by human liver cytosolic glutathione S-transferases. Cancer Research. 1996;**56**(16):3678-3681

[92] Dirven HA, van Ommen B, van Bladeren PJ. Glutathione conjugation of alkylating cytostatic drugs with a nitrogen mustard group and the role of glutathione S-transferases. Chemical Research in Toxicology. 1996;**9**(2): 351-360

[93] Oakley AJ et al. The glutathione conjugate of ethacrynic acid can bind to human pi class glutathione transferase P1-1 in two different modes. FEBS Letters. 1997;**419**(1):32-36

[94] Axarli I et al. Directed evolution of glutathione transferases towards a selective glutathione-binding site and improved oxidative stability. Biochimica et Biophysica Acta (BBA)-General Subjects. 2017;**1861**(1):3416-3428

[95] Zhang K, Wong KP. Glutathione conjugation of chlorambucil: Measurement and modulation by plant polyphenols. Biochemical Journal. 1997; **325**(2):417-422

[96] Hellou J, Ross NW, Moon TW. Glutathione, glutathione S-transferase, and glutathione conjugates, complementary markers of oxidative stress in aquatic biota. Environmental Science and Pollution Research. 2012; **19**(6):2007-2023

[97] Dekant W, Vamvakas S, Anders M. Bioactivation of hexachlorobutadiene by glutathione conjugation. Food and Chemical Toxicology. 1990;**28**(4):285-293

[98] Englert C et al. Crossing the blood-brain barrier: Glutathione-conjugated poly (ethylene imine) for gene delivery. Journal of Controlled Release. 2016;**241**: 1-14

[99] Tephly TR. Isolation and purification of UDP-glucuronosyltransferases. Chemical Research in Toxicology. 1990; **3**(6):509-516

[100] Naritomi Y et al. Prediction of hepatic and intestinal glucuronidation using in vitro–in vivo extrapolation. Drug Metabolism and Pharmacokinetics. 2015;**30**(1):21-29

[101] Wu W et al. In vitro glucuronidation of five rhubarb anthraquinones by intestinal and liver microsomes from humans and rats. Chemico-Biological Interactions. 2014; **219**:18-27

[102] Xing H et al. An investigation on glucuronidation metabolite identification, isozyme contribution, and species differences of GL-V9 in vitro and in vivo. Molecules. 2019; **24**(8):1576

[103] Meng F et al. Identification of human UDP-glucuronosyltransferase isoforms involved in the isofraxidin glucuronidation and assessment of the species differences of the reaction. Fitoterapia. 2017;**117**:118-125

[104] Hong X et al. In vitro glucuronidation of wushanicaritin by liver microsomes, intestine microsomes and expressed human UDP-glucuronosyltransferase enzymes. International Journal of Molecular Sciences. 2017;**18**(9):1983

[105] Nakajima M et al. Imipramine N-glucuronidation in human liver microsomes: Biphasic kinetics and characterization of UDP-glucuronosyltransferase isoforms. Drug Metabolism and Disposition. 2002; **30**(6):636-642

[106] Meech R, Mackenzie PI. Structure and function of uridine diphosphate glucuronosyltransferases. Clinical and Experimental Pharmacology and Physiology. 1997;**24**(12):907-915

[107] Fisher MB et al. In vitro glucuronidation using human liver microsomes and the pore-forming peptide alamethicin. Drug Metabolism and Disposition. 2000;**28**(5):560-566

[108] Irshaid YM, Tephly TR. Isolation and purification of two human liver UDP-glucuronosyltransferases. Molecular Pharmacology. 1987;**31**(1):27-34

[109] Fujiwara R, Yoda E, Tukey RH. Species differences in drug glucuronidation: Humanized UDP-glucuronosyltransferase 1 mice and their application for predicting drug glucuronidation and drug-induced toxicity in humans. Drug Metabolism and Pharmacokinetics. 2018;**33**(1):9-16

[110] Liu H et al. Glucuronidation of macelignan by human liver microsomes and expressed UGT enzymes: Identification of UGT1A1 and 2B7 as the main contributing enzymes. Biopharmaceutics & Drug Disposition. 2014;**35**(9):513-524

[111] Slovak J, Mealey K, Court M. Comparative metabolism of mycophenolic acid by glucuronic acid and glucose conjugation in human, dog, and cat liver microsomes. Journal of Veterinary Pharmacology and Therapeutics. 2017;**40**(2):123-129

[112] Street CM et al. Bisphenol-a glucuronidation in human liver and breast: Identification of UDP-glucuronosyltransferases (UGTs) and influence of genetic polymorphisms. Xenobiotica. 2017;**47**(1):1-10

[113] Hanioka N et al. Glucuronidation of 4-tert-octylphenol in humans, monkeys, rats, and mice: An in vitro analysis using liver and intestine microsomes. Archives of Toxicology. 2017;**91**(3):1227-1232

[114] Zhang X et al. Metabolism of kurarinone by human liver microsomes and its effect on cytotoxicity. Pharmaceutical Biology. 2016;**54**(4):619-627

[115] Wang L et al. Glucuronidation of icaritin by human liver microsomes, human intestine microsomes and expressed UDP-glucuronosyltransferase enzymes: Identification of UGT1A3, 1A9 and 2B7 as the main contributing enzymes. Xenobiotica. 2018;**48**(4):357-367

[116] Cho PJ et al. Identification of specific UGT1A9-mediated glucuronidation of licoricidin in human liver microsomes. Biopharmaceutics & Drug Disposition. 2019;**40**(2):94-98

[117] Jiamboonsri P et al. In vitro glucuronidation of methyl gallate and pentagalloyl glucopyranose by liver microsomes. Drug Metabolism and Pharmacokinetics. 2016;**31**(4):292-303

[118] Miners JO et al. Predicting human drug glucuronidation parameters: Application of in vitro and in silico modeling approaches. Annual Review of Pharmacology and Toxicology. 2004;**44**: 1-25

[119] Kuehl GE et al. Glucuronidation of nonsteroidal anti-inflammatory drugs: Identifying the enzymes responsible in human liver microsomes. Drug Metabolism and Disposition. 2005;**33**(7): 1027-1035

[120] Linnet K. Glucuronidation of olanzapine by cDNA-expressed human UDP-glucuronosyltransferases and human liver microsomes. Human Psychopharmacology: Clinical and Experimental. 2002;**17**(5):233-238

[121] Krishnaswamy S et al. Serotonin (5-hydroxytryptamine) glucuronidation in vitro: Assay development, human liver microsome activities and species differences. Xenobiotica. 2003;**33**(2): 169-180

[122] Gao R et al. Identification and characterization of human UDP-glucuronosyltransferases responsible for the in vitro glucuronidation of ursolic acid. Drug Metabolism and Pharmacokinetics. 2016;**31**(4):261-268

[123] Lv X et al. Glucuronidation of bavachinin by human tissues and expressed UGT enzymes: Identification of UGT1A1 and UGT1A8 as the major contributing enzymes. Drug Metabolism and Pharmacokinetics. 2015;**30**(5):358-365

[124] Maul R et al. In vitro glucuronidation kinetics of deoxynivalenol by human and animal microsomes and recombinant human UGT enzymes. Archives of Toxicology. 2015;**89**(6):949-960

[125] Kirkwood LC, Nation RL, Somogyi AA. Glucuronidation of dihydrocodeine by human liver microsomes and the effect of inhibitors. Clinical and Experimental Pharmacology and Physiology. 1998;**25**(3–4):266-270

[126] Miksits M et al. Glucuronidation of piceatannol by human liver microsomes: Major role of UGT1A1, UGT1A8 and UGT1A10. Journal of Pharmacy and Pharmacology. 2010;**62**(1):47-54

[127] Fuhrmann GF, Völker B. Misuse of graphical analysis in nonlinear sugar transport kinetics by Eadie-Hofstee plots. Biochimica et Biophysica Acta (BBA)-Biomembranes. 1993;**1145**(1): 180-182

Chapter 8

Use of Statins in Dental Implantology and Their Impact on Osseointegration: Animal Studies

Tomislav Katanec and Dragana Gabrić

Abstract

Statins are one of the most commonly used drugs for the prevention of atherosclerosis and ischemic heart disease. Statins have an antibacterial effect against oral pathogens, especially against *Aggregatibacter actinomycetemcomitans* and *Porphyromonas gingivalis*. Studies on animals that we analyzed in this chapter show that statins promote angiogenesis and osteoblast differentiation. Data on the effect of statins on the process of osseointegration are important in clinical practice and should be an integral part of dental education. PubMed, Cochrane Central, and Web of Science database search was performed for animal studies on statin effects on dental osseointegration. Fifteen studies performed on laboratory animals were identified where statins were applied systemically, locally, orally, subcutaneously, or intraosseously. Titan implants of different diameters were placed in tibia and femur of animals. Statins improved osseointegration and enhanced contact of implant surface with the newly formed bone, as well as significantly increased the volume of newly formed bone in lab animals. The purpose of this chapter is to prove the relationship between local use of statins and better osseointegration, as well as a larger amount of newly formed bone around the implant. Knowledge of the effect of frequently prescribed medications on dental procedures and osseointegration is necessary for both students and physicians.

Keywords: statins, osseointegration, dental implants, bone and implant contact, bone metabolism

1. Introduction

Atherosclerosis and ischemic heart disease are the most common causes of death in the world. Hyperlipidemia is one of the most important risk factors for the development of diseases of the cardiovascular system. Prevention and treatment are based on lowering the serum concentration of atherogenic lipoproteins and triglycerides. Statins are one of the most commonly used drugs for this purpose. As structural analogs, they inhibit cholesterol synthesis in liver cells by inhibiting the enzyme 3-hydroxy-3-methylglutaryl-CoA (HMGCoA) reductase. People treated with statins generally continue with this therapy for the rest of their lives. Statins consumption is on the rise and in some countries, those drugs can be bought without a prescription [1].

Statins are rapidly absorbed and the maximum plasma concentration is within 4 hours [2]. The optimal time to take a statin is in the evening before bedtime when the synthesis of endogenous cholesterol is most intense [3]. They are metabolized largely by cytochrome P450 (CYP450). This metabolic pathway is particularly important for lipophilic statins that are highly susceptible to oxidative reactions at cytochrome P450 [4]. Elimination after metabolization in the liver is done mainly by bile. Therefore, hepatic dysfunction is a risk factor for statin-induced myopathy. Hydrophilic statins that bypass the metabolic pathway *via* cytochrome P450 are excreted largely unchanged by the liver and kidneys.

Statins are generally well tolerated and serious side effects are very rare. Mild and transient side effects that may occur include bloating, constipation, diarrhea, abdominal pain, general weakness, and dizziness [5].

Caution should be exercised with regard to dental procedures in patients receiving warfarin therapy because statins may increase the concentration of warfarin in plasma and dose adjustment of warfarin is sometimes required [6]. It is important to note that macrolides, although rarely prescribed in dental clinics, can increase plasma statin concentrations and consequently cause myopathy. It is recommended that statins are discontinued during macrolide therapy if treatment with another group of antibiotics is not possible [7].

Statins have an antibacterial effect against oral pathogens, especially against *Aggregatibacter actinomycetemcomitans* and *Porphyromonas gingivalis* [8]. They also have an antifungal effect against *Candida albicans*, *Aspergillus fumigatus*, and Zygomycetes. Statins modulate the immune response to inflammation and sepsis and reduce the CRP inflammatory parameter by reducing the level of inflammatory interleukin 6. They also increase the level of bone morphogenic protein-2 (BMP-2), stimulate osteoblast activity in bone matrix formation, and promote osseointegration of dental implants [9, 10]. There are several factors that may influence implant and osseointegration such as type of implant-abutment connection. Menini et al. do research on internal versus external connections. They measured peri-implant marginal bone level (MBL) changes, plaque index (PI), probing depth (PD), and bleeding on probing (BoP), evaluated at implant insertion and at 3, 6, and 12 months post-loading. After 12 months, both implant connections showed good clinical features, without inflammation or bone resorption [11]. Animal studies have shown that simvastatin promotes angiogenesis, osteoblast differentiation, and periodontal ligament cell development in both topical and systemic administrations. Angiogenesis and fibrinogenesis are prompted by stimulation of vascular endothelial growth factor (VEGF) in a not yet fully elucidated way [12, 13]. Studies in the United States have shown that more than one-third of the adult population over the age of 45 use systemic statin therapy, putting these drugs in a position to be used as essential therapeutics in dentistry, especially in oral surgery, dental implantology, and periodontology [14].

2. Materials and methods of search strategy

2.1 Literature search strategy

The keywords used in the web search were: (1) statins + osseointegration; (2) statins + implants; (3) statins + implants + osseointegration; (4) BIC + statins; (5) BIC + statins + osseointegration; (6) simvastatin + osseointegration; (7) simvastatin +

implants; (8) rosuvastatin + osseointegration + implants; (9) fluvastatin + osseointegration; and (10) fluvastatin + implants (**Figure 1**).

Keywords were entered into PubMed, Cochrane Central, and Google Scholar databases. The search inclusion criteria were published studies from the creation of the databases to the end of April 2021. Articles that do not have English abstract with the following keywords were eliminated: statins + endodontics, statins + pulpitis, statins + direct pulp coverage, and statins + stem cells. This was done by reviewing the reference list of included articles to identify the potential of an acceptable study. *In vitro* studies investigating oral and perioral microorganisms found in the oral cavity were included in the review. Studies published in languages other than English language were included only if an abstract was available in English. Studies inclusion criteria in this systematic review were if they met the following eligibility

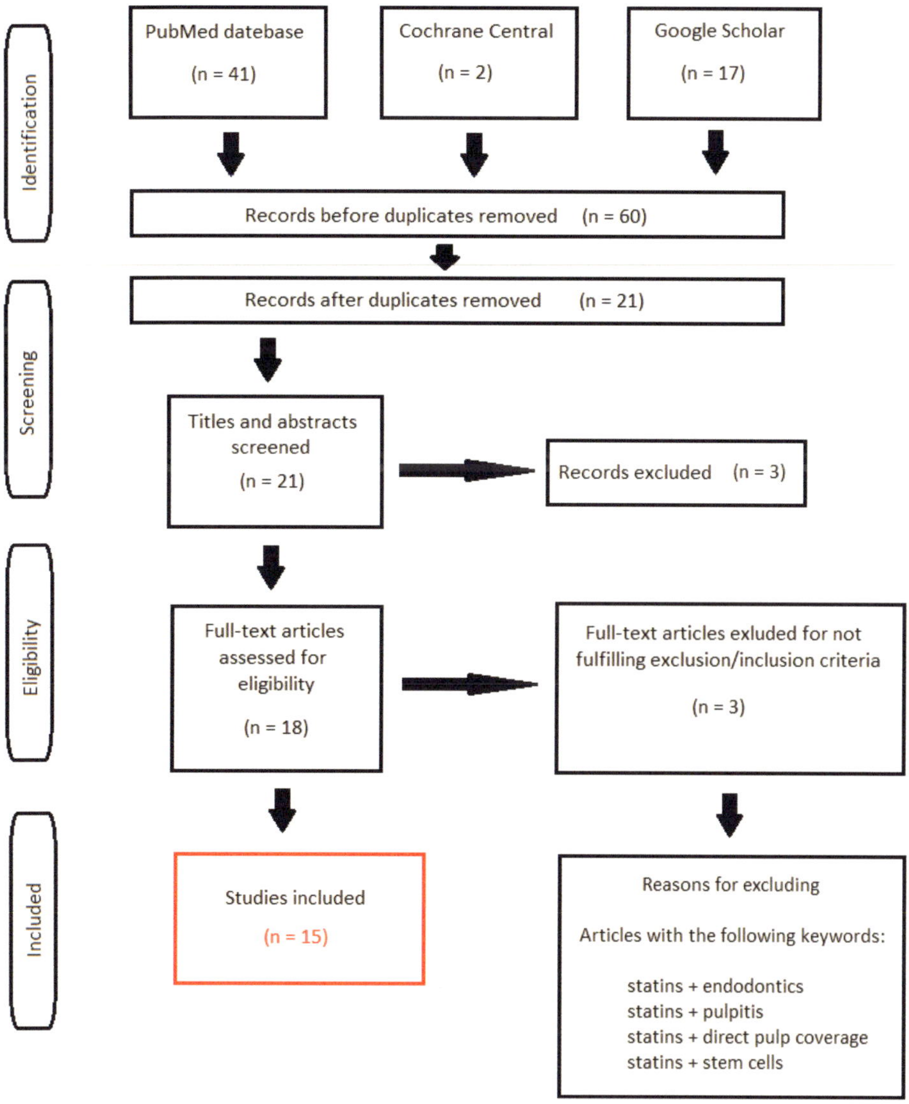

Figure 1.
Flowchart of article selection process in the review.

criteria: original studies in English (clinical and animal trials); evaluation of titanium implants influenced by statins; the presence of a control group; and outcome data considering bone implant contact (BIC), mechanical tests, or other histological evaluation. Studies exclusion criteria was articles using implants inserted into the medullar cavity, Letters to the editor, reviews, case series, case reports, and *in vitro* studies were also exclusion criteria for this chapter.

2.2 Review and identification of acceptable studies

In the initial phase, one author reviewed abstracts of all papers to identify the studies that could have the inclusion criteria. If the abstract met the inclusion criteria, then the full text of the paper was obtained, evaluated, and cited in the review paper. The second author checked all the listed works and the criteria for inclusion or exclusion of certain articles.

3. Effects of statins in animal studies literature review

A total of 60 articles were found. When duplicates and those that did not meet the criteria were excluded, there were 15 publications left that were included in the research.

Table 1 shows the results of this review. A total of 15 papers were included in the analysis. In seven studies, statins were shown to increase the formation of new bone. In two studies, statins promoted better osseointegration of dental implants and in one, there were no significant differences. In five studies, use of statins led to improved contact between the bones and the surface of the implant, and in three

Authors	Test subjects	Number of implants	Implant site	Implant used	Statins: type and dosage	Results
Kellesarian, Al Amri, Al-Kheraif, Ghanem, Malmstrom, Javed [14]	19 laboratory animals: 13 female rats, 1 male rat, 5 dogs of unspecified gender	-	-	Titanium	Simvastatin (per os, s.c., i.o.): 0.25 and 50 mg/kg/day; fluvastatin: 3–300 µg	Better osseointegration and better contact of implant surface with newly formed bone
Fang, Zhao, He, Liu, Yang [15]	36 female rats	72	Distal tibia	Titanium 4 × 2.2 mm	Simvastatin HA surface coat of 1 implant (10^{-7} M and 10^{-6} M)	Increased formation of new bone, better BIC
Kwon, Yang, Lee [16]	3 male rabbits	16	Tibia, femoral head	Titanium 3.5 × 8 mm	Simvastatin 535 µg, surface of 1 implant	Significantly larger volume of newly formed bone and better contact of implant
Faraco-Schwed, Mangueira, Ribeiro, Antao Ada, Shibli [17]	16 male rabbits	32	Tibia	Titanium 3.25 × 8.5 mm	Simvastatin gel 0.25 mg/mL and 30 mg/mL, topically to bone	Significantly better contact of implant after 4 and 8 weeks

Authors	Test subjects	Number of implants	Implant site	Implant used	Statins: type and dosage	Results
Mansour, Al Ashwah, Koura [18]	10 dogs	20	Mandible	Titanium 3.5 × 10 mm	Simvastatin 150 mg topically on 1 implant	Significantly higher volume of newly formed bone
Nyan, Hao, Miyahara, Noritake, Rodriguez, Kasugai [19]	24 male rats	36	Tibia	Titanium 1.8 × 5 mm	Simvastatin 25 and 50 μg to surface of 1 implant	Significantly larger volume of newly formed bone, better contact of newly formed bone and implant surface, larger volume of mineralized newly formed bone
Pauly, Back, Kaeppler, Haas, Schmidmaier, Wildemann [20]	80 female rats	80	Femur	Titanium 1.4 × 5 mm	Simvastatin 5.5 and 90 μg to surface of 1 implant	Significantly larger volume of newly formed bone and better contact of implant surface and newly formed bone, significantly better contact of implant
Yang, Song, Guo, Zhao, Liu, He [21]	48 male rats	96	Tibia	Titanium 2.2 × 4 mm	Simvastatin 10^{-6} M and 10^{-7} M to surface of 1 implant	Histomorphometric analysis showed significantly larger volume of newly formed bone and better implant surface contact with newly formed bone
Moriyama, Ayukawa, Ogino, Atsuta, Koyano [22]	60 rats	60	tibia	Titanium 1 × 1.5 mm	Fluvastatin 3 and 75 μg, simvastatin 15 μg topically on surface of 1 implant	Larger volume of newly formed bone; no significant difference in BIC
Moriyama, Ayukawa, Ogino, Atsuta, Todo, Takao et al. [23]	126 female rats	126	Tibia	Titanium 1 × 1.5 mm	Fluvastatin 3 μg (group 3), 15 μg (group 4), 75 μg (group 5), 300 μg (group 6) topically on surface of 1 implant	Volume of newly formed bone lower in group 6 in comparison to other groups after week 1; volume of newly formed bone and BIC larger in group 5 in comparison to other groups after week 2

Authors	Test subjects	Number of implants	Implant site	Implant used	Statins: type and dosage	Results
Ayukawa, Okamura, Koyano [24]	30-week-old female rats	20	Both tibia	Titanium 1 × 1.5 mm	Experimental group was intraperitoneally administered 10 mg/kg of simvastatin, control group received the isotonic saline instead	In both group newly formed bone was seen to be in direct contact with the implant surface; however, unmineralized connective tissue, including fibroblast-like cells and blood vessels, was occasionally seen on implant surface in experimental group
Xu, Shi, Xu, et al. [25]	30 male rats	30	Maxilla	Titanium implants, diameter 0.8 mm	Oral simvastatin group-25 mg/kg simvastatin, the local simvastatin group-0.8 mg/ 0.05 ml simvastatin around the implant every day	Bone tissue was markedly higher with local simvastatin administration relative to oral simvastatin administration
Jun, Oh, Park, Jung, Li, Moon [26]	12 rabbits	48	Both tibia	Titanium, diameter 3.1 mm	Group C: implants placed without any treatment in rabbits Group U: implants irradiated with UV immediately before implantation, but not coated with simvastatin Group S: implants immersed in simvastatin solution for 24 h in separate sealed containers without UV exposure in rabbits Group SU: implants first immersed in simvastatin solution for 24 h and then irradiated with UV immediately before surgery in rabbits	Ultraviolet (UV) or SIM treatment of SLA titanium implants accelerates osseointegration in tibias with or without xenogenic bone graft materials. The combination of both treatments did not show synergy

Authors	Test subjects	Number of implants	Implant site	Implant used	Statins: type and dosage	Results
Dundar, Bozoglan [27]	16 female rats	16	Tibia	Titanium 2.5 × 4 mm	Test group (8)-5 mg of simvastatin was applied to the bone sockets control group-no simvastatin	No statistically significant differences in ratios of the test group and control group in terms of implant osseointegration ($p > 0.05$)
Apostu, Lucaciu, Mester, Oltean-Dan, Gheban, Rares Ciprian Benea [28]	80 female rats	80	Femur	Titanium Ti90Al6V4 alloy nails	Group I (ovariectomy); Group II (sham ovariectomy); Group III (alendronate 3 mg/kg twice a week + ovariectomy); Group IV (simvastatin 5 mg/kg daily + ovariectomy); and Group V (tibolone 5 mg/kg daily + ovariectomy)	Tibolone could offer the best results in a way of osseointegration

Table 1.
A total of 15 papers that were included in the analysis with their number of test subjects, number of implants that were placed in the study, place where implant was inserted, surface of implant and dosage used in each animal research, and final conclusion of each study.

studies, less mobility of the implant could be demonstrated. In two studies, there were no significant differences in contact between bone and implant, regardless of the statin use.

One study demonstrated more bone formation if simvastatin was administered topically than systemically orally. Tibolone also showed good results in osseointegration compared to simvastatin.

Kellesarian et al. [15] reviewed studies performed on 19 laboratory animals in which simvastatin was administered systemically and locally, specifically orally, subcutaneously, and intraosseously. Better osseointegration and better contact of the implant surface with the newly formed bone were demonstrated in the simvastatin group. A total of 13 studies were performed on female rats, 1 study was on male rats, and 5 studies were performed on dogs of indeterminate sex. Statins were used topically in 12 studies, statins were applied directly to bone cavities in five studies and they were applied systemically in two studies. The dose of systemically administered statins was between 0.25 and 50 mg/kg/day. In two studies, propylene glycol and fluvastatin were used at a dose of 3–300 μg and were applied to the bone bed of the implant before implant placement. Titanium implants were used in all studies.

Studies by Fang et al., Kwon et al., and Faraco-Schwed et al. [16–18] reported that the total number of implants placed in subjects ranged between 16 and 96 implants per research. The total number of implants utilized was not reported in 14 studies. Implants were placed in the tibia and femur in 13 and in 4 studies, respectively. In a study by Kwon et al., 16 implants were placed in the tibia and femur [17]. Fang et al. in their research study work on 36 female rats divided into 3 groups. In the first group, the surface of implants implanted in the tibia is covered with a mixture of hydroxylapatite and simvastatin in the amount of SIM 10^{-7} M (M = 1 mol/liter), in the second group, the surface of implants is covered with the same combination only in the amount of 10^{-6} M, and in the third group, only hydroxylapatite is applied on the surface of implants. Histomorphometric analysis was performed after 2, 4, and 12 weeks and better contact of the newly formed bone with the implant surface was found as well as a higher volume of newly formed bone in the first two groups as opposed to the third group [16]. Kwon et al. performed the research on 3 male rabbits, divided into three groups. A total of 16 implants measuring 3.5 × 8 mm are placed in the tibia and femur. The first group is control and implants are placed without additional surface treatment. In the second group, implants surface is coated only with hydroxylapatite and in the third group, implants surface is covered with hydroxylapatite and simvastatin and a concentration of 535 μg.

Follow-up after 4 weeks was done by micro-CT analysis and biomechanical examination during which a significantly higher volume of newly formed bone and less implant mobility were observed in the third group [17]. Faraco-Schwed et al. conducted a study in which they topically administered statins to 16 male rabbits divided into 4 groups. They used 32 titanium implants implanted in the tibia measuring 3.25 × 8.5 mm. The first group received 0.25 mL of simvastatin gel (30 mg/mL) topically over 28 days, the second group over 56 days, while the third and fourth groups represented the control group. Biomechanical control after 4 and 8 weeks showed significantly less mobility in the second group compared to the fourth, while in the first and third groups there were no statistically significant differences [18].

Mansour et al. studied 10 dogs that received titanium implants in the mandible measuring 3.5 × 10 mm. The duration of the study was 18 months. The first group received simvastatin 150 mg topically *via* implant surface and the second group was the control. Histological analysis of the preparation after 4 and 12 weeks showed a significantly higher amount of newly formed bone in the first compared with the control group [19].

Nyan et al. used 24 male rats divided into 6 groups. The first group was the control. The second group used implants where the surface was treated only by the micro-oxidation technique, while the third group used implants where the surface was treated with micro-oxidation and coated with simvastatin (SIM) in the amount of SIM 25 μg and in the fourth group, the amount of simvastatin used to cover the surface of implants was 50 μg. Micro-CT analysis and histological analysis were performed after 2 and 4 weeks and the results showed significantly higher volume of newly formed bone, better contact of newly formed bone, and implant surface as well as a larger volume of mineralized newly formed bone. Titanium implants measuring 1.8 × 5.0 mm were implanted in the animals' tibia [20].

Pauly et al. divided 80 female rats into 4 groups. The first group was control, while the second group used implants where the surface was treated only with poly D, l-lactide acid (PDDLA) and the third and fourth groups used PDLLA + simvastatin 5.5 μg and PDLLA + simvastatin 90 μg per implant surface. Histological and biomechanical analysis after 8 weeks showed a significantly higher volume of newly formed bone as well as better contact between the surface of the implant and the newly formed bone and significantly less mobility of the implant in the third and fourth groups. Titanium implants measuring 1.4 × 5 mm implanted in the femur were used in the study [21].

Yang et al. implanted 96 titanium implants in a total of 48 female rats with removed ovaries. The implants measured 2.2 × 4.0 mm. The first group underwent ovariectomy, while rats in the other two groups underwent ovariectomy and the surface of implants was coated with a concentration of simvastatin 10^{-7} M for the first group and in the second group with 10^{-6} M. Histomorphometric analysis after 1, 2, 4, and 12 weeks showed a significantly higher volume of newly formed bone and better contact of the implant surface with the newly formed bone in the first two groups [22].

Moriyama et al. conducted their two studies on a total of 186 female rats. The first study was conducted on 60 rats divided into 5 groups that received titanium implants measuring 1 × 1.5 mm in the tibia. Throughout all five groups, authors combined different amounts of propylene glycol alginate (PGA) and fluvastatin (FLU) at different concentrations topically across the implant surface. The first group was the control, while the second group received only PGA, the third group topically received PGA and FLU 3 μg on the surface of the implant, the fourth group received PGA + SIM 15 μg on the surface of implant, and the fifth group received PGA and FLU 75 μg on the surface of the implant. Histomorphometrically, group 5 showed a significantly higher volume of newly formed bone compared to other groups, while there was no significant difference in the quality of contact between the implant surface and the newly formed bone in all five groups. The second study was performed on 126 female rats divided into 6 groups, 21 subjects each. The first group subjects did not receive any topical statin administration and it formed the control group. The second group received topically only PGA, the third group received FLU in the amount of 3 μg; the fourth group received FLU 15 μg, the fifth group FLU 75 μg, and the sixth group received FLU in the amount of 300 μg on the surface of the implant. All animals had titanium implants measuring 1 × 1.5 mm in the tibia. After the first week, the volume of the newly formed bone was lower in group six compared to other groups and after the second week, the volume of newly formed bone and bone contact with the implant was higher in the fifth group compared to other groups [23, 29].

In their review paper, Moraschini et al. [30] also summarize and analyze similar studies as Kellesarian et al. The discussion explained the mechanism of action of statins on the process of osseointegration. Authors concluded that statins enhanced the action of bone-morphogenic protein-2 (BMP-2) which in turn acted on enhanced osteoblastic activity and the formation of new bone. Authors further claimed that in the above studies in which FLU was used in rats, no changes were observed in the form of an increase in the liver enzymes alanine aminotransferase (ALT) or aspartate aminotransferase (AST). The higher the dose used in the studies, the greater the volume of newly formed bone and better seal of newly formed bone and implant surface in the first 2 weeks, which was evident in the study by Moriyama et al.

Türer et al. divided 32 rats into 4 groups: group C-14 (control), group R-14, group C-28 (control), and group R-28. Each animal underwent a unilateral, standard vertical osteotomy on the right side of the mandible, extending from the tooth to the mandibular base. Sterile saline absorbent collagen sponge was applied to the fracture area in groups C-14 and C-28, while an absorbent collagen sponge with saline containing 1 mg rosuvastatin was applied to the fracture area in groups R-14 and R-28. Animals in groups C-14 and R-14 were euthanized on day 14 and the animals in groups C-28 and R-28 were euthanized on day 28 after surgery. Stereological analyses were performed. New areas of bone and connective tissue volume were measured. Stereological analysis showed that the R-14 group had significantly more new bone after 2 weeks compared to the C-14 group. The volume of connective tissue was also significantly higher in R-14. Differences in connective tissue volume and new bone were not statistically significant upon comparison of groups C-28 and R-28. Topically applied rosuvastatin enhanced early bone regeneration in rats with mandibular fracture [31].

Keuroghlian et al. investigated mice with the assumption that hyperlipidemia negatively affected the osseointegration of dental implants because a high-fat diet had significant detrimental effects on bone density and volume. The authors placed a group of male mice on a high-fat diet and a control group on a regular diet. After 12 weeks, every animal received a titanium implant in the femur. Animals were humanely sacrificed 4 or 8 weeks after implantation, and the results showed that a high-fat diet significantly reduced bone density and strength and that osseointegration was poorer [32].

The work of Mahrous, who investigated the topical application of simvastatin in gel form for the treatment of peri-implant mucositis, was found in the Cochrane Central database. The author tested the proven anti-inflammatory effect of statins on the inflamed mucosa surrounding dental implants. The hypothesis was that 1.2% of simvastatin gel would reduce inflammation around the implant. The pilot study involved 44 subjects divided into a test and a control group. The test group received topically simvastatin gel that was applied with a blunt-tipped needle around the implant while thc control group received a placebo. The inflammatory condition was determined at the beginning of the study, 24 hours later, after 1 week, and after 1 month by clinical indications for inflammation and biochemical markers of inflammation collected around the implant. The study included individuals of both sexes who had no signs of bone resorption around the implant by more than 1 mm as established by X-ray analysis. The results showed that the greatest reduction in inflammation occurred in the first 24 hours, but there were no statistically significant differences in the levels of cytokines IL-1β, IL-6, IL-8, and TNF-α between the test and control group as well as no significant differences in periodontal probing depth [24].

Ayukawa et al. performed the animal study on 10 female rats that were 30 weeks old. Ten titanium implants were placed in both tibias and measured 1 mm in diameter and 1.5 mm in length. Experimental group received intraperitoneally 10 mg/kg of simvastatin, and the control group received isotonic saline instead. Both groups showed that the newly formed bone was thought to be in direct contact with the implant surface. Despite direct contact of the new bone and implant surface, the experimental group showed occasional evidence of unmineralized connective tissue, including fibroblast-like cells and blood vessels, on implant surface [25].

Rongyao Xu et al. performed implants in oral cavity on 30 male rats that were postoperatively randomly divided into three groups. The first group received 25 mg/kg of simvastatin orally, the second group received simvastatin injections in the amount 0.8 mg/0.05 mL around the implant every day, and the third group was the control. Simvastatin promoted osseointegration of the implant. Rats that were treated with simvastatin had more newly formed bone that had a woven appearance than control group rats as revealed by H&E staining. In addition to that, the volume of bone tissue was significantly higher in rats that received simvastatin locally in comparison with the group that received simvastatin orally [26].

Hoon Yun et al. researched the effect of ultraviolet (UV) and simvastatin (SIM) treatment on the osseointegration of dental titanium implants in rabbit tibias at two different time points. Implants were sandblasted, large-grit, and acid-etched (SLA) and surface alterations due to simvastatin treatment were analyzed with an infrared spectrometer. Implants were divided into four groups depending on the type of surface treatment of implants. Twelve rabbits were implanted with two implants per tibia. Implants were in contact with the surface of the bone and bovine bone was used as graft material for gap filling. Animals were humanely sacrificed after 2 or 4 weeks. Results showed that bone-to-implant contact (BIC) was increased with UV treatment and SIM immersion on non-grafted sides and both BIC and bone area (BA) were increased on grafted sides. BIC or BA did not increase with both treatments in comparison with a single treatment. As data were collected at two different time points, results showed that BIC in the non-grafted sides did not differ significantly among UV- and/or SIM-treated groups, but BA was significantly different among groups. Ultraviolet or simvastatin treatments on SLA titanium implants accelerated osseointegration in tibias with or without xenogenic bone graft materials. Joint implementation of both treatments did not show significant positive effects [27].

Dundar and Bozoglan conducted their research on 16 female rats during a 4-week experimental trial. The subject was divided into two groups: a test group (n = 8) that received local simvastatin and a control group (n = 8) that did not receive simvastatin treatment. A titanium implant was surgically implanted into the tibial metaphysis of all 16 animals. Ethanol solution in the amount of 100 μl containing 5 mg simvastatin was applied to the bone sockets before implantation. Results for bone-implant contact (BIC) showed no statistically significant differences among test and control groups with regard to implant osseointegration ($p > 0.05$) [28].

Apostu et al. evaluated and compared the effects of different treatments (simvastatin, alendronate, and tibolone) on improved osseointegration of titanium implants. Research was conducted on 80 female albino Wistar rats evenly divided into five groups: Group 1 underwent ovariectomy, group 2 underwent false ovariectomy, group 3 underwent ovariectomy and alendronate treatment, group 4 underwent ovariectomy and simvastatin treatment, and group 5 underwent ovariectomy and tibolone treatment. Three months post-ovariectomy, the authors performed bilateral titanium intramedullary nailing (Ti90A16V4 alloy nails) in all groups followed by a 12-week oral administration of alendronate (3 mg/kg twice a week), simvastatin (5 mg/kg daily), or tibolone (5 mg/kg daily). Micro CT, mechanical pull-out test, histology, and bone serum markers were examined after 12-week oral treatment. Upon review of all examination results, the authors concluded that the initial hypothesis that simvastatin, alendronate, and tibolone enhance osseointegration in ovariectomized rats with intramedullary titanium implants has been accepted. Tibolone showed the best results out of three treatments [33].

4. Pharmacokinetics of simvastatin

The chemical structure of all statins consists of the pharmacophore and its moiety containing a ring system with different substituents. The pharmacophore is shared among all statins, and it is a dihydroxyheptanoic acid segment that is very similar to the HMGCoA substrate [34]. The ring system consists of a complex hydrophobic structure covalently linked to the pharmacophore and it is involved in binding interactions with the HMG-CoA reductase enzyme [35]. There are different kinds of statins, which differ from each other in their hydrophobic ring structure and its substituents, covalently linked to the HMG-like moiety. These differences in structure affect the pharmacological properties of the statins [36].

The lipophilicity of the statins is considered important since the hepatoselectivity of the statins is related to their degree of lipophilicity. The higher the lipophilicity of statins, the greater level of exposure it gets to non-hepatic tissues, while the more hydrophobic statins have a tendency to be more selective for the liver, whereas lipophilic statins passively and nonselectively diffuse into both hepatocytes and non-heptatocytes. The more hydrophobic statins largely rely on active transport into hepatocytes to exert their effects [37].

There are two forms of statins, lactone (inactive) and open-ring hydroxy acid (active) forms. The HMG-like moiety that all statins are in the inactive form as a lactone. Simvastatin and lovastatin are administered as lactone prodrugs and subsequently transformed into active metabolites. The remaining statins become in their active form as a β-hydroxy acid. *In vivo*, lactone statins are hydrolyzed to their hydroxy acid pharmacophores in the liver to achieve pharmacological activity [38].

We can divide statins into two groups: naturally or fungal-derived (type 1) and synthetic (type 2). One of the main differences between the type 1 and type 2 statins is the replacement of the fluorophenyl group of type 2 statins with the butyryl group in type 1 statins. These specific groups cause additional polar interactions and stronger and tighter binding to the HMGR enzyme. Functionally, the methylethyl group attached to the central ring of the type 2 statins replaces the decalin of the type 1 statins. The butyryl group of the type 1 statins occupies a region similar to the fluorophenyl group present in the type 2 inhibitors [39].

The hepatoselectivity is very important factor in liposolubility of the statins and their inhibitory effect on HMG-CoA reductase. Lipophilic statins enter the hepatocytes through passive diffusion, whereas hydrophilic statins undergo a carrier-mediated membrane [40].

Hydrophilicity depends on a transport process that takes the drug from the portal blood into hepatocytes using anion-transporting polypeptides (OATP). That molecules give better potential and selectivity for the liver cells. Hydrophilic statins—such as rosuvastatin and pravastatin—have higher potential to the liver metabolism, because they harder way of entering other tissues as lipophilic statins do. However, the balance between desired and undesired effects of lipophilic and hydrophilic statins remains not clearly established [41].

5. Effect of statin on bone metabolism

The bone tissue is a very dynamic formation that is always remodeled by bone cells osteoclasts and bone-forming osteoblasts.

Osteoblast cells are derived from mesenchymal stem cells and osteocytes derived from terminally differentiated osteoblasts [42, 43].

The biggest amount of lipids is present in bone marrow, and the lowest concentration of them in bone mineral matrix. Human bone contains 28–84% of neutral lipids, and only less than 3% of phospholipids [44].

Cholesterols have function in bone metabolism, in which membrane signal transducing platforms and play crucial roles in RANK-RANKL signal transduction during osteoclastogenesis.

High cholesterol levels also increase bone metabolism. High fat diets in mice caused osteoclastogenesis, and decrease in bone mass. The high-fat-fed antigen-induced arthritis (AIA) model also suggested that enhanced cathepsin K-positive osteoclasts contributed to more severe deterioration of the joints than in normal-diet-fed AIA rabbits [45–47].

Cellular cholesterol has important role in cellular metabolism of macrophages pathways. Macrophages have the same origin as osteoclasts. The low-density lipoprotein receptor (LDLR) on macrophages promotes the internalization of ApoB-containing lipoprotein, resulting in high levels of intracellular cholesterol [48, 49].

Osteoporosis is an epidemic throughout the world and is associated with trauma fractures in the vertebral spine, femoral neck, and distal radius. Specifically, post-menopausal osteoporosis is connected with pathological bone fractures. That is very often a disease in elderly women. It is typically associated with low bone mass and poor bone density.

Bisphophonates, selective estrogen receptor modulators, calcitonin, and vitamin D analogues are most usefully drugs for osteoporosis. They can also stop further bone loss. All of these drugs are inhibitors of bone resorption that act mainly to stabilize bone mass. It is hard to say if they are also osteoinductive [50, 51].

Osteoporosis and atherosclerosis share the tendency to accelerate after menopause; both diseases are promoted by inflammatory processes, and many aspects of arterial calcification and bone formation are similar [52]. The relationship between osteoporosis and atherosclerosis is supported by the observation that the progression of aortic calcification is most severe in women with the most severe metacarpal bone loss. Factors that may promote both processes include estrogen deficiency and increased concentrations of proinflammatory cytokines, such as IL-1, IL-6, and TNF-a [49, 50].

6. Conclusion

A review of the results from the available literature shows that statins have a future in the use within oral surgery procedures and implantology where their osteogenic effect is most pronounced and their influence on the increase of the volume of newly formed bone and contact between implants and bone. Although studies have been conducted on small animals we believe that the potential of statins in bone formation is also high in humans. One of the studies also demonstrated the effectiveness of statins on bone fracture regeneration. We believe that local use of a statin applied to the bone bed of the implant, as well as topical application of a liquid statin to the implant surface, shows better osseointegration potential of the implant, as well as better contact of the implant with the more newly formed bone. A better effect on the soft tissues around the implant is also visible. It is possible that local statins increase level of bone morfogenic protein-2 (BMP-2) in bone metabolism, which affects higher level of newly formed bone. Future studies should establish safe and effective clinical protocols for statin application to promote osseointegration.

Conflict of interest

The authors declare that there is no conflict of interest.

Author details

Tomislav Katanec[1,2]* and Dragana Gabrić[1,2]

1 Department of Oral Surgery, School of Dental Medicine, University of Zagreb, Zagreb, Croatia

2 Department of Oral Surgery, University Hospital Centre Zagreb, Zagreb, Croatia

*Address all correspondence to: tkatanec@sfzg.hr

References

[1] Kaufman DW, Kelly JP, Rosenberg L, Anderson TE, Mitchell AA. Recent patterns of medication use in the ambulatory adult population of the United States: The Slone survey. Journal of the American Medical Association. 2002;**287**(3):337-344

[2] Igel M, Sudhop T, von Bergmann K. Metabolism and drug interactions of 3-hydroxy-3-methylglutaryl coenzyme A-reductase inhibitors (statins). European Journal of Clinical Pharmacology. 2001;**57**(5):357-364

[3] Schachter M. Chemical, pharmacokinetic and pharmacodynamic properties of statins: An update. Fundamental & Clinical Pharmacology. 2005;**19**(1):117-125

[4] Bottorff M, Hansten P. Long-term safety of hepatic hydroxymethyl glutaryl coenzyme A reductase inhibitors: The role of metabolism-monograph for physicians. Archives of Internal Medicine. 2000;**160**(15):2273-2280

[5] Nigović B, Fabijanić P, Bačić-Vrca V. Statini. Farmaceutski Glasnik. 2007;**63**(5):315-331

[6] Grau E, Perella M, Pastor E. Simvastatin-oral anticoagulant interaction. Lancet. 1996;**347**(8998): 405-406

[7] Grunden JW, Fisher KA. Lovastatin-induced rhabdomyolysis possibly associated with clarithromycin and azithromycin. The Annals of Pharmacotherapy. 1997;**31**(7-8):859-863

[8] Emani S, Gunjiganur GV, Mehta DS. Determination of the antibacterial activity of simvastatin against periodontal pathogens, *Porphyromonas gingivalis* and *Aggregatibacter actinomycetemcomitans*: An in vitro study. Contemporary Clinical Dentistry. 2014;**5**(3):377-382

[9] Ting M, Whitaker EJ, Albandar JM. Systematic review of the in vitro effects of statins on oral and perioral microorganisms. European Journal of Oral Sciences. 2016;**124**(1):4-10

[10] Mundy G, Garrett R, Harris S, et al. Stimulation of bone formation in vitro and in rodents by statins. Science. 1999;**286**(5446):1946-1949

[11] Menini M, Pesce P, Bagnasco F, Carossa M, Mussano F, Pera F. Evaluation of internal and external hexagon connections in immediately loaded full-arch rehabilitations: A within-person randomised split-mouth controlled trial. International Journal of Oral Implantology (Berlin). 2019;**12**(2):169-179 PMID: 31090748

[12] Henwood JM, Heel RC. Lovastatin. A preliminary review of its pharmacodynamic properties and therapeutic use in hyperlipidaemia. Drugs. 1988;**36**(4):429-454

[13] Todd PA, Goa KL. Simvastatin. A review of its pharmacological properties and therapeutic potential in hypercholesterolaemia. Drugs. 1990;**40**(4):583-607

[14] Wang HE, Griffin R, Shapiro NI, Howard G, Safford MM. Chronic statin use and long-term rates of sepsis: A population-based cohort study. Journal of Intensive Care Medicine. 2014;**31**(6):386-396

[15] Kellesarian SV, Al Amri MD, Al-Kheraif AA, Ghanem A,

Malmstrom H, Javed F. Efficacy of local and systemic statin delivery on the osseointegration of implants: A systematic review. The International Journal of Oral & Maxillofacial Implants. 2017;**32**(3):497-506

[16] Fang W, Zhao S, He F, Liu L, Yang G. Influence of simvastatin-loaded implants on osseointegration in an ovariectomized animal model. BioMed Research International. 2015;**2015**:831504

[17] Kwon YD, Yang DH, Lee DW. A titanium surface-modified with nano-sized hydroxyapatite and simvastatin enhances bone formation and osseintegration. Journal of Biomedical Nanotechnology. 2015;**11**(6):1007-1015

[18] Faraco-Schwed FN, Mangueira LM, Ribeiro JV, Antao Ada S, Shibli JA. Removal torque analysis of implants in rabbit tibia after topical application of simvastatin gel. The Journal of Oral Implantology. 2014;**40**(1):53-59

[19] Mansour G, Al Ashwah A, Koura A. Evaluation of simvastatin grafting around immediate dental implants in dogs. Implant Dentistry. 2014;**23**(2):195-199

[20] Nyan M, Hao J, Miyahara T, Noritake K, Rodriguez R, Kasugai S. Accelerated and enhanced bone formation on novel simvastatin-loaded porous titanium oxide surfaces. Clinical Implant Dentistry and Related Research. 2014;**16**(5):675-683

[21] Pauly S, Back DA, Kaeppler K, Haas NP, Schmidmaier G, Wildemann B. Influence of statins locally applied from orthopedic implants on osseous integration. BMC Musculoskeletal Disorders. 2012;**13**:208

[22] Yang G, Song L, Guo C, Zhao S, Liu L, He F. Bone responses to simvastatin-loaded porous implant surfaces in an ovariectomized model. The International Journal of Oral & Maxillofacial Implants. 2012;**27**:369-374

[23] Moriyama Y, Ayukawa Y, Ogino Y, Atsuta I, Koyano K. Topical application of statin affects bone healing around implants. Clinical Oral Implants Research. 2008;**19**:600-605

[24] Mahrous AM. Use of topical subgingival application of simvastatin gel in the treatment of peri-implant mucositis [Master's Thesis]. Graduate College, The University of Iowa Iowa City, Iowa. 2018

[25] Ayukawa Y, Okamura A, Koyano K. Simvastatin promotes osteogenesis around titanium implants. Clinical Oral Implants Research. 2004;**15**(3):346-350

[26] Xu R, Shi G, Xu L, et al. Simvastatin improves oral implant osseointegration via enhanced autophagy and osteogenesis of BMSCs and inhibited osteoclast activity. Journal of Tissue Engineering and Regenerative Medicine. 2018;**12**:1209-1219

[27] Jun JH, Oh KC, Park K-H, Jung N, Li J, Moon HS. Improvement of osseointegration by ultraviolet and/or simvastatin treatment on titanium implants with or without bone graft materials. Materials. 2021;**14**(13):3707

[28] Dundar S, Bozoglan A. Evaluation of the effects of topically applied simvastatin on titanium implant osseointegration. Journal of Oral Biology and Craniofacial Research. 2020;**10**(2):149-152

[29] Moriyama Y, Ayukawa Y, Ogino Y, Atsuta I, Todo M, Takao Y, et al. Local application of fluvastatin improves periimplant bone quantity and mechanical properties: A rodent study. Acta Biomaterialia. 2010;**6**:1610-1618

[30] Moraschini V, Almeida DCF, Calasans-Maia JA, Calasans-Maia MD. The ability of topical and systemic statins to increase osteogenesis around dental implants: A systematic review of histomorphometric outcomes in animal studies. International Journal of Oral and Maxillofacial Surgery. 2018;**47**:1070-1078

[31] Türer A, Durmuşlar MC, Şener I, Misir AF, Önger ME. The effect of local rosuvastatin on mandibular fracture healing. The Journal of Craniofacial Surgery. 2016;**27**(8):758-761

[32] Keuroghlian A, Viana Barroso AD, Kirikian G, Bezouglaia O, Tintut Y, Tetradis S, et al. The effects of hyperlipidemia on implant osseointegration in the mouse femur. The Journal of Oral Implantology. 2015;**41**(2):7-11

[33] Apostu D, Lucaciu O, Mester A, Oltean-Dan D, Gheban D, Benea H. RC. Tibolone, alendronate and simvastatin enhance implant osseointegration in a preclinical in vivo model. Clinical Oral Implants Research. 2020 Jul;**31**(7):655-668

[34] Stancu C, Sima A. Statins: Mechanism of action and effects. Journal of Cellular and Molecular Medicine. 2001;**5**:378-387

[35] Gazzerro P, Proto MC, Gangemi G, Malfitano AM, Ciaglia E, Pisanti S, et al. Pharmacological actions of statins: A critical appraisal in the management of cancer. Pharmacological Reviews. 2012;**64**:102-146

[36] Roche VF. Teachers' topics: Antihyperlipidemic statins: A self-contained, clinically relevant medicinal chemistry lesson. American Journal of Pharmaceutical Education. 2005;**69**:546-560

[37] Pfefferkorn JA, Song Y, Sun KL, Miller SR, Trivedi BK, Choi C, et al. Design and synthesis of hepatoselective, pyrrole-based HMG-CoA reductase inhibitors. Bioorganic & Medicinal Chemistry Letters. 2007;**17**:4538-4544

[38] Corsini A, Maggi FM, Catapano AL. Pharmacology of competitive inhibitors of HMG-CoA reductase. Pharmacological Research. 1995;**31**:9-27

[39] Istvan ES, Deisenhofer J. Structural mechanism for statin inhibition of HMG-CoA reductase. Science. 2001;**292**:1160-1164

[40] Hamelin BA, Turgeon J. Hydrophilicity/lipophilicity: Relevance for the pharmacology and clinical effects of HMG-CoA reductase inhibitors. Trends in Pharmacological Sciences. 1998;**19**:26-37

[41] Whirl-Carrillo M, McDonagh EM, Hebert JM, Gong L, Sangkuhl K, Thorn CF, et al. Pharmacogenomics knowledge for personalized medicine. Clinical Pharmacology and Therapeutics. 2012;**92**:414-417

[42] Feng X, McDonald JM. Disorders of bone remodeling. Annual Review of Pathology. 2011;**6**:121-145

[43] Eriksen EF. Cellular mechanisms of bone remodeling. Reviews in Endocrine & Metabolic Disorders. 2010;**11**:219-227

[44] Lund PK, Abadi DM, Mathies JC. Lipid composition of normal human bone marrow as determined by column chromatography. Journal of Lipid Research. 1962;**3**:95-98

[45] Ryu J, Kim H, Chang EJ, Kim HJ, Lee Y, Kim HH. Proteomic analysis of osteoclast lipid rafts: The role of the integrity of lipid rafts on V-ATPase activity in osteoclasts. Journal of Bone and Mineral Metabolism. 2010;**28**:410-417

[46] Lee YD, Yoon SH, Park CK, Lee J, Lee ZH, Kim HH. Caveolin-1 regulates osteoclastogenesis and bone metabolism in a sex-dependent manner. The Journal of Biological Chemistry. 2015;**290**:6522-6530

[47] Prieto-Potin I, Roman-Blas JA, Martinez-Calatrava MJ, Gomez R, Largo R, Herrero-Beaumont G. Hypercholesterolemia boosts joint destruction in chronic arthritis. An experimental model aggravated by foam macrophage infiltration. Arthritis Research & Therapy. 2013;**15**:R81

[48] Moore KJ, Sheedy FJ, Fisher EA. Macrophages in atherosclerosis: A dynamic balance. Nature Reviews. Immunology. 2013;**13**:709-721

[49] Sato T, Morita I, Murota S. Involvement of cholesterol in osteoclast-like cell formation via cellular fusion. Bone. 1998;**23**(2):135-140

[50] Lips P. Epidemiology and predictors of fractures associated with osteoporosis. The American Journal of Medicine. 1997;**103**(2A):3S-11S

[51] Riggs BL, Hartmann LC. Selective estrogen-receptor modulators – mechanisms of action and application to clinical practice [published correction appears in *The New England Journal of Medicine* 2003;348(12):1192]. The New England Journal of Medicine. 2003;**348**(7):618-629

[52] Tintut Y, Demer LL. Recent advances in multifactorial regulation of vascular calcification. Current Opinion in Lipidology. 2001;**12**(5):555-560

Section 4

Drugs and Doses

Chapter 9

Perspective Chapter: Tuberculosis Drugs Doses from Indian Scenario – A Review

Pooja Pawar, Inampudi Sailaja and Ivvala Anand Shaker

Abstract

Tuberculosis is an infectious disease spread through the air that is treated with a combination of drugs. Compliance to long-term antituberculosis therapy is vital for sustaining adequate blood drug level. Inadequate medical management of patients is a major factor in the emergence and dissemination of drug-resistant Mycobacterium TB strains. The necessity to understand the context of individual and collective health when considering tuberculosis treatment remains a difficulty. Furthermore, when it comes to treatment success, social and economic factors have been demonstrated to be aspects that must be considered. Because of the poor, expensive, ineffective, and toxic alternatives to first-line medications, the therapeutic approach for drug-resistant tuberculosis is complicated. New antituberculosis medications (bedaquiline and delamanid) have recently been licenced by health authorities; however, they do not constitute a definitive answer for the clinical management of drug-resistant tuberculosis forms, especially in middle-income countries where drug resistance is common (China, India, and former Soviet Union countries). There is an immediate need for new research and development initiatives. To sustain both new and ancient therapeutic choices, public health policies are essential. We did a thorough review of national and international literature on tuberculosis treatment in India in recent years with the goal of providing advice to health care providers based on the scenario.

Keywords: tuberculosis, drug-resistant, mycobacterium, antituberculosis, medications, health policies

1. Introduction

Tuberculosis (TB) continues to have a major influence on global healthcare. For more than five decades, anti-tubercular treatment (ATT) is available but still, about one-third of the world's population continues to be infected with tuberculosis [1]. In the last decade, the rise of multidrug-resistant tuberculosis (MDR-TB) and extensively drug-resistant tuberculosis (XDR-TB) has sparked global alarm [1–3]. Patients who are infected with strains resistant to isoniazid and rifampicin, called multidrug-resistant (MDR) TB, are practically incurable by standard first-line treatment (Seung et al. 2015).

Tuberculosis (TB) is a global health concern that causes 8.7 million new cases and 1.4 million deaths each year [4]. Furthermore, resistant *Mycobacterium tuberculosis* strains are appearing in practically all places reported to the World Health Organisation (WHO) [5]. Noncompliance with treatment regimens and incorrect TB therapy prescriptions are thought to be key contributors to this public health issue [6, 7]. Fixed-dose combination (FDC) tablets, each combining two or more anti-TB drugs, have been manufactured since the 1980s [8] to simplify TB therapy and facilitate physician and patient compliance with treatment recommendations [9] due to the large number of tablets used in TB treatment regimens. These Fixed-dose combination (FDC) pills also avoid unintended monotherapy, which can happen due to prescription errors, insufficient regimens, or patient error in taking only one medicine [10]. Furthermore, dealing with a single combined formulation including all needed medications streamlines drug procurement, storage, and delivery, potentially lowering drug supply management errors and costs. The World Health Organisation (WHO) and the International Union Against Tuberculosis and Lung Disease (IUATLD) approved FDC anti-TB therapy in 1994 [11]. Concerns were raised about adequate bioavailability of the component drugs following the announcement of this recommendation and its more widespread implementation, particularly rifampicin (RIF) due to its enhanced decomposition in the presence of isoniazid (INH) [12, 13]. As a result, the WHO and the IUATLD set bioavailability standards for FDC anti-TB medication components [14]. Two-drug formulations (INH + RIF and INH + ethambutol), three-drug formulations (INH + RIF + ethambutol and INH + RIF + pyrazinamide), and a four-drug formulation (INH + RIF + ethambutol + pyrazinamide) are currently on the WHO Model List of Essential Drugs [10, 15].

The first three years of implementation of the National Strategic Plan (2017–2025) to eradicate tuberculosis in India have been completed. The programme has had a lot of success over this time [16]. Through the NIKSHAY portal, the initiative has made significant progress toward near-complete online notification of all TB cases in the country. The system has notified 24.04 lakh patients, an increase of 11% over previous year, with 6.7 lakh patients from the private sector being notified. For 22.7 lakh (94.4%) of the declared drug-sensitive TB cases, first-line standard treatment was started. Early case discovery has improved as a result of mapping high-risk groups, properly planned systematic screening, and aggressive case finding for active TB, resulting in lower transmission risks, poor treatment outcomes, and negative social and economic implications. This year, 27.74 crore people were examined in 337 districts across 23 states, yielding 62,958 TB cases [16].

Tuberculosis (TB) is a disease that has been around for a long time. Despite the availability of tubercle bacillus chemotherapy, our fight against this ancient human foe is far from ended. Because of the pathogen's peculiar biological properties [17]. Springett [18] describes the disease as having a distinct natural history and a sluggish response to currently available chemotherapeutic treatments [17, 19, 20]. Since the beginning of chemotherapy, poor treatment adherence, developed drug resistance, treatment failure, and relapse have all been reported [21]. A series of seminal experiments in Madras (now Chennai), Africa, Hong Kong, and Singapore led to create the now widely used 6-month standard regimens administered under supervision [22]. These research set the groundwork for the World Health Organisation's (WHO) global comprehensive TB control strategy, known as directly observed therapy, short-course (DOTS), which was announced in 1993 alongside a proclamation of tuberculosis as a global emergency [23]. Despite some recent debates on the exact importance of the act of directly observed treatment (DOT) [24, 25], no other mode of drug administration has been shown to provide a comparable high rate of treatment success as DOTS in functional programme settings [26]. Since the introduction of DOTS, intermittent drug delivery has been frequently used to facilitate treatment oversight on an outpatient basis, either throughout the 6-month course or solely during the continuation phase in the last 4 months [21]. The fewer treatment visits reduces both operational and patient-related costs, particularly when extensive travel distances are involved. Patients can go about their daily routines and work as usual because intermittent treatment has a lower impact on their everyday lives [21]. This facilitates patient access to therapy and treatment adherence, particularly in resource-constrained places or for underserved groups [21]. The scientific basis for intermittent TB treatment in clinical settings has been established by in vitro evidence of the post-antibiotic effect (PAE), which showed that exposure to medicines, particularly isoniazid, for a few hours resulted in suppression of mycobacterial growth for several days [27, 28]. The free peak drug concentration to minimum inhibitory concentration (MIC) ratio best correlates with the PAE and resistance suppression for rifampicin and perhaps other TB treatments [21, 28].

2. Current status in India

The persistence of an immune response to *M. tuberculosis* antigen stimulation without any clinically active disease is known as latent tuberculosis infection (LTBI) [29]. LTBI is expected to affect roughly one-third of the world's population [30]. There are no estimates of the frequency of LTBI in the general population in India; however, according to WHO data, around 3.5 lakh children under the age of five years were eligible for LTBI treatment [31]. Although the majority of infected people do not show symptoms, they are at high risk of developing active infection and so serve as a bacterium reservoir. Reactivation of tuberculosis is believed to be 5–10% of the time [32]. This risk is substantially higher in HIV-positive people, who face a 10% annual risk of reactivation, and in young children (10%). If left untreated, 40% of LTBI children under the age of one develop active disease, compared to 24 per cent in children aged one to ten years and 16% in children aged eleven to fifteen years [33]. Infected people are thought to congregate in a pool of LTBI, from which those with latent TB emerge with active TB. The size of the pool of latent infection must be reduced in order to regulate the active infection [32, 34].

The elimination of tuberculosis (TB) has received a lot of attention in recent decades. While treating active disease is by far the most significant intervention, LTB treatment is an important but underestimated component. The cost of testing, a lack of consensus on the tests that should be used, and treatment side effects all make it difficult to diagnose and treat LTBI [32]. Treatment of LTBI in low-prevalence (high- to upper-middle-income) countries is possible, as removing the infection reservoir reduces the disease's burden. In high-prevalence countries like India, however, the situation is completely different [32]. Here, rather than reactivation, reinfection due to contact with current cases contributes to a high disease burden. This is why there is no national policy on the treatment of LTBI. In this case, LTBI treatment must be tailored to the person [32]. Those at high risk of reactivation should be given priority, especially when the predisposing condition is reversible in the short term. As a result, the probability of reactivation vs. reinfection should be considered while deciding whether or not to treat LTBI [32].

3. Multi-drug-resistant tuberculosis and RNTCP

Tuberculosis (TB) continues to be a major global public health issue that requires immediate response. There are three separate but overlapping components to current global efforts to control tuberculosis: humanitarian, public health, and economic. The main humanitarian concern for a patient-centred approach to TB control is to reduce TB-related sickness, suffering, and mortality. To reduce disease transmission, the public health dimension focuses on correct identification and treatment of patients with tuberculosis. This involves the creation of well-structured tuberculosis control programmes (responsive and adaptable to the reforming health sector). The advent of medication resistance to treat tuberculosis, particularly multidrug-resistant tuberculosis (MDR TB), has become a major public health issue and a roadblock to successful TB control [2]. In the presence of pharmaceuticals, drug resistance manifests itself as a selective expansion of resistant mutants among the actively growing bacillary population. The prevalence of drug resistant mutants in the susceptible bacillary population, the size of the actively growing bacillary population in the lesions, and the antimicrobial quality of the medications utilised all influence the formation of drug resistance [35, 36].

4. Fixed-dose combination antituberculosis therapy

The World Health Organisation and the International Union Against Tuberculosis and Lung Disease (IUATLD) endorsed FDC anti-TB therapy in 1994 [11]. Concerns were raised about proper bioavailability of the component medications following the release of this proposal and its more widespread application, particularly rifampicin (RIF) due to its accelerated breakdown in the presence of isoniazid (INH) [12, 13]. Despite the potential benefits of FDC anti-TB medicines, questions about their efficacy remain unanswered. Many observational studies and clinical trials have been done to determine the efficacy of FDC medications in preventing treatment failure, illness relapse, and drug resistance. The use of FDC medications has resulted in favourable [37], unfavourable [38], or no therapy outcomes in various investigations [39, 40]. Despite current conflicting findings, the WHO [41], the International Standards for Tuberculosis Care (Standard 8) [42], and the American Thoracic Society all endorse FDC formulations for active TB treatment [10, 43].

5. Treatment of latent tuberculosis infection in India

Because it can sterilise latent infection, LTBI chemotherapy is the sole biological TB control intervention. Isoniazid, at a dose of 10 mg/kg/day for 6 months, is suggested by the IAP for the treatment of LTBI. The following people should receive treatment:

- Regardless of their TST, BCG, or nutritional state, asymptomatic contacts (under 6 years of age) of a smear-positive case who have no evidence of active disease should be administered in.
- After screening out active TB, all HIV positive children in contact with an infectious TB case or TST positive (5 mm induration).
- Immunosuppression was planned for or received by TST positive children (e.g., acute leukaemia and nephrotic syndrome).

- If there is no evidence of congenital TB in the new-born child born to a TB positive mother [44].

In adults, individuals with RA and LTBI who are scheduled for immunosuppression should be treated (biologicals). This is in accordance with the ACR's recommendations [45]. Chemotherapy is started in HIV patients as stated above. However, because there are no defined rules for India, therapy for immunocompromised people and close contacts of active cases is done on a case-by-case basis. In nations with a high incidence of tuberculosis, treatment options include isoniazid monotherapy for 6 months, rifampicin and isoniazid combination daily for 3 months (in children 15 years), and rifapentine and isoniazid weekly for 3 months. Isoniazid is administered to adults at a dose of 5 mg/kg and to children at a dose of 10 mg/kg up to a maximum of 300 mg. When utilised, rifampicin is administered at a dose of 10 mg/kg for adults and 15 mg/kg for children, with a maximum dose of 600 mg [31]. All of the following regimens were shown to be non-superior in the majority of studies undertaken to date. However, some regimens may be favoured over others on a case-by-case basis. Rifapentine/rifampicin-containing regimens, for example, are not recommended for HIV patients due to the significant risk of medication interactions. In some cases, these may be preferable because they are shorter and patients are more likely to comply. However, the financial ramifications must also be considered [32].

6. Surgical treatment of tuberculosis

Although tuberculosis is usually treated with drugs, it can also be treated surgically in select situations, particularly in cases of drug resistance and some pulmonary tuberculosis sequelae. Surgical lung biopsy can be used to distinguish between pulmonary tuberculosis and lung cancer. Endobronchial tuberculosis, as well as significant adverse responses, severe haemoptysis, empyema, pneumothorax, and bronchopleural fistula, are all surgical indications. Surgical intervention may be indicated in situations of symptomatic pulmonary residual, fungal ball, and haemoptysis in tuberculosis sequelae [46, 47].

7. Treatment services under national TB elimination programme in India

The National Tuberculosis Elimination Program (NTEP) aims to reach every TB patient for free diagnosis and treatment. In 2019, 94% of TB patients who had been notified were started on treatment for the disease [16]. According to current policy, universal DST is supplied to informed TB patients (including private sector TB patients) to determine the presence of Rifampicin resistance at the time of TB diagnosis in order to provide an appropriate regimen based on the Drug Susceptibility Test (DST). Further tests are offered based on the DST result, as part of the integrated DR TB methodology, to rule out resistance to additional medications. UDST was offered to 58% of all reported TB patients in 2019 [16]. As a result of DST, suitable changes in the regimen are made in accordance with the PMDT standards in India [16].

7.1 Treatment of drug sensitive TB

When a patient is diagnosed with tuberculosis, a standard first-line anti-TB regimen in the form of Fixed Dosage Combination (FDC) is given to them right away, usually from the centre where the diagnosis was made or while the patient is being transferred to the appropriate health facility for treatment initiation, especially when the diagnosis is not the same as the TB patient's relapse (e.g. Mobile or migrant population). The NIKSHAY digital surveillance system enables for the tracking of tuberculosis patients who are referred or transferred from one health unit to another across multiple geographic locations. Through several means, including the PPSA, the National TB Elimination Program has expanded free access to anti-TB drugs to patients seeking care in the private sector. The National TB Elimination Programme uses the services of a contact centre to provide patient counselling and connect them with suitable public resources for patients who are unaware of the nearest diagnostic or therapy institution [16].

7.2 Programmatic Management of Drug Resistant TB services (PMDT)

PMDT services were first offered in 2007, and by 2013, the programme had expanded to encompass the entire country. During 2011–2012, a systematic approach to scaling up all of these facilities was implemented, with coordinated efforts from numerous stakeholders resulting in national coverage by 2013. Line Probe Assay (LPA) was first presented in 2009, followed by CBNAAT in 2012, and both technologies have now been scaled up to 64 LPA labs, 1180 CBNAAT sites, and 350 TrueNAT sites by the end of 2019. By implementing Guidelines for PMDT in India 2017, DRTB treatment services are delegated to district DRTB centres with the goal of bringing drug resistant TB treatment closer to TB patients' homes. By the end of 2019, 711 DR TB centres, including 154 Nodal DR TB centres, will be operational, allowing for decentralised DR-TB treatment. This decentralisation will enable districts to use the "test and treat approach" to shorten diagnostic and treatment delays, reduce travel costs, and speed early MDR/RR-TB patient care within their district [16].

8. Drugs for tuberculosis

As the disease has refused to go away over the previous five decades, there has always been a need for innovative medications and combinations. Many medications are in various stages of development and are being tested. Efforts are being made to produce newer medications, as well as newer regimens that use these drugs [1].

8.1 New applications of existing drugs

8.1.1 Rifamycins

Rifampicin, Rifabutin, and Rifapentine are among the medications in this class. It has been proposed that a greater dose of Rifampicin than the standard 10 mg/kg may be required to reduce treatment duration in new tuberculosis patients. Some mouse trials have provided promising findings in evaluating the role of high-dose rifampicin (15–30 mg/day) in the intense phase of ATT [40]. For the first two months of ATT, a phase II randomised trial comparing rifampicin in dosages of 20 mg/kg/day and 15. mg/kg/day to the usual 10 mg/kg/day is continuing [48]. Preliminary research suggests that greater dosages of Rifampicin are tolerated well, with proportionately higher serum concentration levels [49]. Adults have also been given higher doses of Rifampicin as part of a regular ATT regimen, as well as when combined with other newer medications like Moxifloxacin and SQ-109 [50]. With such high rifampicin doses, there is the potential for a shorter treatment duration, according to current findings. Rifabutin is often preferred over Rifampicin for individuals with TB and HIV since it has fewer medication interactions and negative effects [51]. In children, the dose is 5 mg/kg, while in adults, it is 150–300 mg/day [52].

Rifapentine, another medicine in the same class, has a longer half-life and has been explored for latent tuberculosis infection (LTBI) rather than active tuberculosis. In adults, a three-month preventive regimen of 300 mg Rifapentine and 900 mg Isoniazid was found to be as efficacious as nine months of 300 mg daily Isoniazid [53]. Doses ranging from 300 to 900 mg have been administered in children with adequate tolerance. In order to obtain systemic exposures consistent with successful treatment of LTBI in adults, higher weight-adjusted dosages are required in children [54].

8.1.2 Flouroquinolones

Moxifloxacin and Levofloxacin are the most important medications in this class, and their superiority over other quinolones has been thoroughly established [55]. There have been multiple trials with promising results using quinolones in combination with other first-line medicines to reduce the length of ATT [56]. In the intensive phase, a typical ATT regimen was compared to a Gatifloxacin/Moxifloxacin-containing regimen with the goal of reducing the treatment period to four months, however the latter had greater relapse rates than the former. Furthermore, children under the age of five are known to clear quinolones from the body more quickly in the urine and have a lower serum concentration than adults. There is a scarcity of pharmacokinetic data, particularly in children under the age of five. As a result, optimising their use in children for the prevention of drug resistance becomes more important [55]. Children's usage of quinolones has traditionally been restricted due to worries of arthropathy, however there is no evidence of such side effects in either children or adults treated with long-term quinolones, according to available data.

8.1.3 Oxazolidinones

This family of medicines works by inhibiting protein synthesis by competing with an enzyme involved in translation [57]. Cycloserine was the first oxazolidinone to be used as an antitubercular medication, although linezolid is now the most widely used. Sputum conversion rates in patients with XDR-TB improved in two recent randomised control trials with linezolid [58]. However, higher failure rates at lower doses (300 mg/day) and more severe adverse effects at higher doses (600 mg/day) limit its long-term use. Common side effects include peripheral neuropathy, gastrointestinal problems, and myelosuppression [59]. Both Cycloserine and Linezolid are currently designated by WHO as core medicines for the treatment of drug-resistant tuberculosis. There is not much information on their use as anti-tubercular agents in youngsters.

8.1.4 Beta-lactams and Macrolides

The medications included in WHO group D for treating drug-resistant tuberculosis are amoxycillin-clavulanate, imipenem-cilastin, and meropenem. Meropenem and Clavulanate show substantial synergistic antibacterial action against M. tuberculosis in vitro because Clavulanate suppresses â-lactamase and increases Meropenem's antibacterial activity [60]. In vitro activity against tuberculosis bacilli was demonstrated in a recent research using a triple therapy consisting of amoxicillin, clavulanate, and meropenem [61]. Macrolides, particularly Clarithromycin, have previously proven beneficial in treating non-tubercular mycobacteria, but the outcomes in M. TB have been poor due to fast resistance development [62].

8.1.5 Newer drugs Bedaquiline

After nearly four decades, the Food and Medicine Administration (FDA) has approved this drug as the first antitubercular agent. It blocks the proton pump, which is essential for ATP generation, as well as the mycobacterium's metabolism [62]. Bedaquiline should only be utilised when the typical MDR regimen cannot be constructed due to in vitro resistance to these medications, known adverse drug reactions, poor tolerance, or contraindications to any of the combination regimen's components. It can only be used as part of second-line ATT in patients over the age of 18 years, according to WHO guidelines. However, in the same dosage as advised for adults, it has been found to be effective and safe in children and adolescents [63]. The dose is 400 mg once a day for two weeks, then 200 mg three times a week for the next 22 weeks, for a total of six months, which is the longest time bedaquiline can be given. The Indian government's Revised National Tuberculosis Control Program (RNTCP) is introducing this medicine through a limited access programme across the country. Nausea, vomiting, dizziness, arthralgia, myalgia, elevated serum amylase and transaminase levels, QT prolongation, and dark urine are all known side effects of bedaquiline. Bedaquiline toxicity is increased by drugs that decrease liver function via CYP3A4 metabolism (e.g., ketoconazole and ritonavir) [64].

8.1.6 Delamanid and pretomanid

Both of these medications are nitroimidazoles, which work by preventing mycobacterial cell wall formation [65]. Delamanid has been investigated significantly more thoroughly than pretomanid. In patients with MDR-TB/XDR-TB who have a high baseline risk for poor outcomes, WHO recommends using delamanid for just six months of rigorous treatment at a dose of 100 mg twice a day [66]. When delamanid was given in combination with an improved background regimen in patients with drug resistant tuberculosis, higher rates of sputum conversion and lower mortality were seen [67]. Pretomanid, on the other hand, is a prodrug that requires bio-reductive activation of an aromatic group in order to be effective against tuberculosis. In an experimental mouse model of tuberculosis, it also showed significant bactericidal activity during both the intense and continuation stages of treatment. In 2016, the World Health Organisation (WHO) published guidelines for the use of delamanid in children and adolescents, stating that children with MDR-TB who are resistant to quinolones or second-line injectables (or both) should be candidates for this treatment. This medicine should be used as an add-on treatment in longer MDR-TB regimens (18–24 months) in children rather than as part of the shorter MDR-TB regimens introduced by WHO in 2016 [3]. Not only has the use of bedaquiline, delamanid, and pretomanid transformed the treatment of drug-resistant tuberculosis, but it has also revolutionised the treatment of HIV-TB coinfection.

8.1.7 Other drugs

SQ-109 is an ethambutol analogue with 1, 2 ethylenediamine. This drug is now being tested in people after showing promising results in both in vitro and in vivo mice models of tuberculosis [68]. With isoniazid, rifampicin, and streptomycin, SQ-109 has been demonstrated to have a synergistic effect. SQ-109 reduces Rifampicin's Minimum Inhibitory Concentration (MIC), and this synergy may be important in patients with Rifampicin-resistant TB [1, 69].

9. Preventive measures of MDR-TB through high quality treatment

Drug-resistant tuberculosis (DR-TB) poses a significant national and international programmatic challenge as well as a significant risk to individuals residing in TB-endemic countries. Only about 30% of the 490,000 people estimated to have developed multidrug-resistant tuberculosis (MDR-TB) (along with an additional 110,000 cases of rifampicin [RMP]-resistant TB) in 2016 had their diagnosis, and only about 25% had their treatment for MDR-TB started, according to the World Health Organisation (WHO) [3, 70].

Although existing drug-resistant cases must also be treated, mathematical modelling reveals that best-practice shortcourse chemotherapy can control isoniazid- or rifampicin-resistant disease while preventing the formation of MDR-TB by obtaining cure rates over 80% in new cases [71]. Focusing on enhanced and quality-controlled bacteriology with universal drug susceptibility testing (DST), quality therapy, removal of healthcare access barriers, and appropriate monitoring and evaluation can avoid the occurrence of MDR-TB in addition to high rates of case-detection and cure (WHO, 2015). This patient-centred strategy is further supported by the International Standards for Tuberculosis Care and its regional variations [72, 73].

Since patients with suspected DR-TB are what drives transmission, the cornerstone of MDR-TB transmission prevention should concentrate on earlier diagnosis and prompt initiation of effective therapy for all DR-TB patients (this includes patients on treatment for DS-TB who have undiagnosed DR-TB as well as those who remain both undiagnosed and untreated) [74]. Making these patients non-infectious will enhance individual outcomes and reduce transmission. A 90% decrease in TB incidence is one of the lofty goals put forth in the WHO's End TB Strategy, which was introduced in 2015 [75]. The End TB Strategy mandates that all individuals being tested for TB, not just those with recognised risk factors for developing DR-TB disease, undergo universal drug susceptibility testing (DST). This method necessitates a large expansion of the use of molecular diagnostics for TB, which allow an early evaluation of treatment resistance at the time of TB diagnosis [70].

Early diagnosis and efficient treatment are essential components of an effective MDR-TB (Multi Drug Resistant Tuberculosis) control approach, similar to DS-TB (Drug Susceptible Tuberculosis). One of the main causes of continued TB transmission is diagnostic delay. Drug susceptibility testing (DST), which is necessary for the diagnosis of drug-resistant tuberculosis (DR-TB), was previously unavailable in the majority of high-prevalence settings until the recent introduction of rapid genotypic DST using GeneXpert MTB/RIF® or Line Probe Assays (such as INNO-LiPA® and Genotype MTBDRsl®) [76]. However, there is still a sizable case detection gap, and it is estimated that in 2014, 75% of MDR-TB patients were unreported [77]. Only 12% of newly diagnosed TB cases with bacteriological confirmation and 58% of TB people who have already received treatment around the world have DST done. The 2016 WHO MDR-TB treatment recommendations include a strong recommendation for universal DST for all TB patients at the time of initial diagnosis [3]. The proposed "F-A-S-T" strategy, which is based on rapid DST (drug susceptibility testing), is designed to find cases actively by cough monitoring and rapid molecular sputum testing, separate securely, and treat efficiently. This improved guidance is applicable to all settings and age categories [78]. Since these techniques will require significant investment from health systems to become a reality, more study is needed to determine their usefulness [79].

10. Another strategy we can follow is prevent transmission through infection control

Effective infection control measures are crucial in clinical facilities that treat TB and M/XDR-TB patients, according to the WHO Policy on Infection Control [71, 80, 81]. The plan of action comprises administrative, environmental, and management controls [73, 77, 81].

It is well recognised that poverty increases M. tuberculosis transmission, TB mortality rates, and TB incidence [71, 82]. Even in wealthy nations, detecting and treating MDR-/XDR-TB can be expensive. However, using new medications may be more affordable [73]. The correct application of modern diagnostic tools and medications, along with the fundamental measures provides the foundation for the prevention and control of MDR-TB [72, 77, 83–89]. Recently, efforts to end TB have concentrated on latent TB infection (LTBI) diagnosis and treatment as well as TB control in risk groups (displaced populations) [71, 73]. To identify LTBI in high risk and vulnerable groups, interferon-gamma release assays (IGRAs) or Mantoux tuberculin skin test (TST) are both advised, while novel regimens comprising rifampicin and rifapentine are currently advised, being especially helpful in isoniazid resistant cases [73]. The majority of TB infections are found among migrants and refugees in various high-income nations, and these populations are the main source of new cases among locals [71, 73]. Those vulnerable groups should have unrestricted access to TB services after moving to a new country, and quick, excellent TB and LTBI management should be ensured. Clinical professionals have a moral obligation to properly manage both drug-susceptible and MDR-TB in order to meet TB elimination targets [73].

11. Conclusion

It is commonly acknowledged that TB management in India will continue to face significant hurdles as long as TB treatment is dominated by such a vast and fragmented private sector. Approaches like the ones discussed here, when combined with already available surveillance techniques, could help to create a comprehensive picture of the state of the private sector, how it develops over time, and where interventions are most needed. Future interventions to harness the private sector for the benefit of TB patients in India and worldwide will benefit greatly from such monitoring.

Author details

Pooja Pawar[1], Inampudi Sailaja[2] and Ivvala Anand Shaker[3*]

1 Department of Microbiology, Parul Institute of Applied Sciences, Parul University, Vadodara, Gujarat, India

2 Department of Biochemistry, Parul Institute of Applied Sciences, Parul University, Vadodara, Gujarat, India

3 Department of Biochemistry, Parul Institute of Medical Sciences and Research, Parul University, Vadodara, Gujarat, India

*Address all correspondence to: ivvala.shaker@paruluniversity.ac.in

References

[1] Khurana AK, Dhingra B. What is new in management of paediatric tuberculosis? Paediatric Tuberculosis Management. 2019;**56**:213-220

[2] TB India 2016. Revised National Tuberculosis Control Programme 2016, Annual Status Report. Available from: http://www.tbcindia.nic.in [Accessed: June 2, 2017]

[3] World Health Organisation. Who Treatment Guidelines for Drug-resistant Tuberculosis. Geneva: WHO; 2016

[4] World Health Organisation (WHO). Global tuberculosis control: WHO report 2012. WHO/HTM/TB/2012.6

[5] World Health Organisation (WHO). Multidrug and extensively drug-resistant TB (M/XDR-TB): 2010 global report on surveillance and response. WHO/HTM/TB/2010.3

[6] Mitchison DA. How drug resistance emerges as a result of poor compliance during short course chemotherapy for tuberculosis. The International Journal of Tuberculosis and Lung Disease. 1998;**2**:10-15

[7] van Altena R, van Soolingen D, van der Werf TS. Isoniazid resistant TB and non-compliance. Thorax. 2004;**59**:1098

[8] Norval PY, Blomberg B, Kitler ME, et al. Estimate of the global market for rifampicin-containing fixed-dose combination tablets. The International Journal of Tuberculosis and Lung Disease. 1999;**3**(Suppl. 3):S292-S300

[9] Bangalore S, Kamalakkannan G, Parkar S, et al. Fixed-dose combinations improve medication compliance: A metaanalysis. The American Journal of Medicine. 2007;**120**:713-719

[10] Albanna AS, Smith BM, Cowan D, Menzies D. Fixed-dose combination antituberculosis therapy: A systematic review and meta-analysis. The European Respiratory Journal. 2013;**42**:721-732

[11] A joint statement of the International Union Against Tuberculosis and Lung Disease and the Tuberculosis Programme of the World Health Organisation. The promise and reality of fixed dose combinations with rifampicin. Tubercle and Lung Disease. 1994;**75**:180-181

[12] Milan-Segovia RC, Domınguez-Ramırez AM, Jung-Cook H, et al. Relative bioavailability of rifampicin in a threedrug fixed-dose combination formulation. The International Journal of Tuberculosis and Lung Disease. 2010;**14**:1454-1460

[13] Shishoo CJ, Shah SA, Rathod IS, et al. Impaired bioavailability of rifampicin in presence of isoniazid from fixed dose combination (FDC) formulation. International Journal of Pharmaceutics. 2001;**228**:53-67

[14] A joint statement of the International Union Against Tuberculosis and Lung Disease and the World Health Organisation. Assuring bioavailability of fixed-dose combinations of anti-tuberculosis medications. The International Journal of Tuberculosis and Lung Disease. 1999;**3**(Suppl. 3): S282-S283

[15] WHO Model List of Essential Medicines. 17th list (March 2011). WHO Drug Information. 2011

[16] Ministry of Health and Family Welfare, India. INDIA TB REPORT. New Delhi: Central TB Division, Ministry of Health and Family Welfare; 2020

[17] Mitchison DA. The search for new sterilising anti-tuberculosis drugs. Frontiers in Bioscience. 2004;**9**:1059e72

[18] Springett VH. Ten-year results during the introduction of chemotherapy for tuberculosis. Tubercle. 1971;**52**:73e87

[19] Mitchison DA. Role of individual drugs in the chemotherapy of tuberculosis. The International Journal of Tuberculosis and Lung Disease. 2000;**4**:796e806

[20] Zhang Y. Advances in the treatment of tuberculosis. Clinical Pharmacology and Therapeutics. 2007;**82**:595e600

[21] Chang KC, Leung CC, Grosset J, Yew WW. Treatment of tuberculosis and optimal dosing schedules. Thorax. 2011;**66**:997-1007

[22] Fox W, Ellard GA, Mitchison DA. Studies on the treatment of tuberculosis undertaken by the British Medical Research Council tuberculosis units, 1946e1986, with relevant subsequent publications. The International Journal of Tuberculosis and Lung Disease. 1999;**3**:S231e79

[23] World Health Organisation. Global Tuberculosis Programme. Global Tuberculosis Control. Geneva, Switzerland: WHO; 1997

[24] Kamolratanakul P, Sawert H, Lertmaharit S, et al. Randomised controlled trial of directly observed treatment (DOT) for patients with pulmonary tuberculosis in Thailand. Transactions of the Royal Society of Tropical Medicine and Hygiene. 1999;**93**:552e7

[25] Walley JD, Khan MA, Newell JN, et al. Effectiveness of the direct observation component of DOTS for tuberculosis: A randomised controlled trial in Pakistan. Lancet. 2001;**357**:664e9

[26] Sharma SK, Liu JJ. Progress of DOTS in global tuberculosis control. Lancet. 2006;**367**:951e2

[27] Chan CY, Au-Yeang C, Yew WW, et al. Postantibiotic effects of antituberculosis agents alone and in combination. Antimicrobial Agents and Chemotherapy. 2001;**45**:3631e4

[28] Gumbo T, Louie A, Deziel MR, et al. Concentration-dependent *M. tuberculosis* killing and prevention of resistance by rifampin. Antimicrobial Agents and Chemotherapy. 2007;**51**:3781e8

[29] Mack U, Migliori GB, Sester M, Rieder HL, Ehlers S, Goletti D, et al. LTBI: Latent tuberculosis infection or lasting immune responses to *M. tuberculosis*? A TBNET consensus statement. The European Respiratory Journal. 2009;**33**:956-973

[30] Dye C, Scheele S, Dolin P, Pathania V, Raviglione MC. Consensus statement. Global burden of tuberculosis: Estimated incidence, prevalence, and mortality by country. WHO Global Surveillance and Monitoring Project. JAMA. 1999;**282**:677-686

[31] WHO. Latent Tuberculosis Infection: Updated and Consolidated Guidelines for Programmatic Management. Geneva: World Health Organisation; 2018

[32] Saha S, Kumar A, Saurabh K, Shanka SH, Kashyap A, Nischal N, et al. Current status of treatment of latent tuberculosis infection in India. Indian Journal of Medical Sciences. 2019;**71**(2):54-59

[33] Health AGD. Tuberculosis (TB). Australian Government Department of Health. 2017. Available from:

http://www.health.gov.au/internet/main/publishing.nsf/content/cdna-songtuberculosis#_ENREF_15 [Accessed: January 10, 2017]

[34] Singh M, Saini AG, Anil N, Aggarwal A. Latent tuberculosis in children: Diagnosis and management. Indian Journal of Pediatrics. 2011;**78**:464-468

[35] Grover GS, Takkar J. Recent advances in multi-drug-resistant tuberculosis and RNTCP. Indian Journal of Community Medicine. 2008;**33**(4):219-223

[36] Smith SE, Pratt R, Trieu L, Barry PM, Thai DT, Ahuja SD, et al. Epidemiology of paediatric MDR tuberculosis in the United States, 1993-2004. Clinical Infectious Diseases. 2017;**16**:1437-1443

[37] Moulding TS, Le HQ, Rikleen D, et al. Preventing drug-resistant tuberculosis with a fixed dose combination of isoniazid and rifampin. The International Journal of Tuberculosis and Lung Disease. 2004;**8**:743-748

[38] Suryanto AA, van den Broek J, Hatta M, et al. Is there an increased risk of TB relapse in patients treated with fixeddose combination drugs in Indonesia? The International Journal of Tuberculosis and Lung Disease. 2008;**12**:174-179

[39] Bartacek A, Schut D, Panosch B, et al. Comparison of a four-drug fixed-dose combination regimen with a single tablet regimen in smear-positive pulmonary tuberculosis. The International Journal of Tuberculosis and Lung Disease. 2009;**13**:760-766

[40] Lienhardt C, Vernon A, Raviglione MC. New drugs and new regimens for the treatment of tuberculosis: Review of the drug development pipeline and implications for national programmes. Current Opinion in Pulmonary Medicine. 2010;**16**:186-193

[41] World Health Organisation (WHO). Treatment of Tuberculosis: Guidelines. 4th ed. Geneva: World Health Organisation; 2009

[42] Tuberculosis Coalition for Technical Assistance. International Standards for Tuberculosis Care (ISTC). 2nd ed. The Hague: Tuberculosis Coalition for Technical Assistance; 2009

[43] American Thoracic Society, CDC, Infectious Diseases Society of America. Treatment of tuberculosis. MMWR Recommended Report. 2003;**52**:1-77

[44] Updated National Guidelines for Paediatric Tuberculosis in India. 2012. Available from: http://www.indianpediatrics.net/mar2013/mar-301-306.htm [Accessed: April 4, 2017]

[45] Singh JA, Saag KG, Bridges SL Jr, Akl EA, Bannuru RR, Sullivan MC, et al. 2015 American college of rheumatology guideline for the treatment of rheumatoid arthritis. Arthritis Care & Research (Hoboken). 2016;**68**:1-25

[46] Conde MB, Melo FA, Marques AM, Cardoso NC, Pinheiro VG, Dalcin Pde T, et al. III Brazilian Thoracic Association Guidelines on tuberculosis. Jornal Brasileiro de Pneumologia. 2009;**35**(10):1018-1048

[47] Rabahi MF, da Silva Júnior JR, Ferreira AG, Tannus-Silva DS, Conde MB. Tuberculosis treatment. Jornal Brasileiro de Pneumologia. 2017;**43**(5):472-486

[48] Milstein M, Lecca L, Peloquin C, Mitchison D, Seung K, Pagano M, et al. Evaluation of high-dose rifampin in

patients with new, smear-positive tuberculosis (HIRIF): Study protocol for a randomised controlled trial. BMC Infectious Diseases. 2016;**16**:453

[49] Peloquin CA, Velasquez GE, Lecca L, Calderon RI, Coit J, Milstein M, et al. Pharmacokinetic evidence from the HIRIF trial to support increased doses of rifampin for tuberculosis. Antimicrobial Agents and Chemotherapy. 2017;**25**(61): e00038

[50] Boeree MJ, Heinrich N, Aarnoutse R, Diacon AH, Dawson R, Rehal S, et al. High-dose rifampicin, moxifloxacin, and SQ109 for treating tuberculosis: A multi-arm, multi-stage randomised controlled trial. The Lancet Infectious Diseases. 2017;**17**:39-49

[51] Horne DJ, Spitters C, Narita M. Experience with rifabutin replacing rifampin in the treatment of tuberculosis. The International Journal of Tuberculosis and Lung Disease. 2011;**15**:1485-1490

[52] Moultrie H, Mcllleron H, Sawry S, Kellerman T, Weisner L, Kindra G, et al. Pharmacokinetics and safety of rifabutin in young HIV infected children receiving rifabutin and lopinavir/ritonavir. The Journal of Antimicrobial Chemotherapy. 2015;**70**:543-549

[53] Sterling TR Villarino ME, Borisov AS, Shang N, Gordin F, Bliven-Sizemore E, et al. Three months of rifapentine and isoniazid for latent tuberculosis infection. The New England Journal of Medicine. 2011;**365**:2155-2166

[54] Weiner M, Savic RM, Kenzie WR, Wing D, Peloquin CA, Engle M, et al. Rifapentine pharmacokinetics and tolerability in children and adults treated once weekly with rifapentine and isoniazid for latent tuberculosis infection. Journal of Paediatric Infectious Diseases. 2014;**3**:132-145

[55] Thee S, Garcia-Prats AJ, Donald PR, Hesseling AC, Schaff HS. Fluroquinolones for the treatment of tuberculosis in children. Tuberculosis (Edinburgh, Scotland). 2015;**95**:229-245

[56] Gillespie SH, Crook AM, McHugh TD, Mendel CM, Meredith SK, Murray SR, et al. Four-month moxifloxacin-based regimens for drug-sensitive tuberculosis. The New England Journal of Medicine. 2014;**371**:1577-1587

[57] Mohan A, Kumar DP, Harikrishna J. Newer Anti-TB Drugs and Drug Delivery Systems. New Delhi: Jaypee Brothers Medical Publishers (for The Association of Physicians of India); 2013. pp. 388-392

[58] Tang S, Yao L, Hao X, Zhang X, Liu G, Liu X, et al. Efficacy, safety and tolerability of linezolid for the treatment of XDR-TB: A study in China. The European Respiratory Journal. 2015;**45**:161-170

[59] Zhang X, Falagas ME, Vardakas KZ, Wang R, Qin R, Wang J, et al. Systematic review and meta-analysis of the efficacy and safety of therapy with linezolid containing regimens in the treatment of multidrug-resistant and extensively drug-resistant tuberculosis. Journal of Thoracic Disease. 2015;**7**:603-615

[60] D'Ambrosio L, Centis R, Sotgiu G, Pontali E, Spanevello A, Migliori GB. New anti-tuberculosis drugs and regimens: 2015 update. ERJ Open Research. 2015;**1**:00010-02015

[61] Gonzalo X, Drobniewski F. Is there a place for â-lactams in the treatment of multidrug-resistant/extensively drug resistant tuberculosis? Synergy

between meropenem and amoxicillin/clavulanate. The Journal of Antimicrobial Chemotherapy. 2013;**68**:366-369

[62] Dooley KE, Obuku EA, Durakovic N, Belitsky V, Mitnick C, Nuermberger EL, et al. World Health Organisation group 5 drugs for the treatment of drug-resistant tuberculosis: Unclear efficacy or untapped potential? The Journal of Infectious Diseases. 2013;**207**:1352-1358

[63] Achar J, Hewison C, Cavalheiro AP, Skrahina A, Cajazeiro J, Nargiza P, et al. Off-label use of bedaquiline in children and adolescents with multidrug resistant tuberculosis. Emerging Infectious Diseases. 2017;**23**:1711-1713

[64] Pontali E, D'Ambrosio L, Centis R, Sotgiu G, Migliori GB. Multidrug-resistant tuberculosis and beyond: An updated analysis of the current evidence on bedaquiline. The European Respiratory Journal. 2017;**22**:49

[65] Xavier AS, Lakshmanan M. Delamanid: A new armour in combating drug-resistant tuerculosis. Journal of Pharmacology and Pharmacotherapeutics. 2014;**5**:222-224

[66] World Health Organisation. The use of bedaquiline in the treatment of multidrug-resistant tuberculosis: Interim policy guidance. 2013. Available from: http://www.who.int/en/ [Accessed: September 6, 2017]

[67] Gupta R, Geiter LJ, Wells CD, Gao M, Cirule A, Xiao H. Delamanid for extensively drug resistant tuberculosis. The New England Journal of Medicine. 2015;**373**:291-292

[68] Chen P, Gearhart J, Protopopova M, Einck L, Nacy CA. Synergistic interactions of SQ109, a new ethylene diamine, with front-line antitubercular drugs in vitro. The Journal of Antimicrobial Chemotherapy. 2006;**58**:332-337

[69] Nikonenko BV, Protopopova M, Samala R, Einck L, Nacy CA. Drug therapy of experimental tuberculosis (TB): Improved outcome by combining SQ109, a new diamine antibiotic, with existing TB drugs. Antimicrobial Agents and Chemotherapy. 2007;**51**:1563-1565

[70] Nathavitharana RR, Lederer P, Tierney DB, Nardell E. Treatment as prevention and other interventions to decrease MDR-TB transmission. The International Journal of Tuberculosis and Lung Disease. 2019;**23**(4):396-404

[71] World Health Organisation. CSV Files, World Health Organisation Latent TB Estimates; 2015a. Available from: http://www.who.int/tb/country/data/download/en. [Accessed: March 20, 2017]

[72] Migliori GB, Zellweger JP, Abubakar I, Ibraim E, Caminero JA, De Vries G, et al. European union standards for tuberculosis care. The European Respiratory Journal. 2012;**39**:807-819

[73] Rendon A, Centis R, D'Ambrosio L, Migliori GB. WHO strategies for the management of drug-resistant tuberculosis. Archivos de Bronconeumología. 2017;**53**(3):95-97

[74] Miller ACLV, Khan FA, Atwood S, Kornienko S, Kononenko Y, Vasilyeva I, et al. Turning off the tap: Using the FAST approach to stop the spread of drug-resistant tuberculosis in Russian Federation. The Journal of Infectious Diseases. 13 Jul 2018;**218**(4):654-658

[75] Uplekar M, Weil D, Lonnroth K, Jaramillo E, Lienhardt C, Dias HM, et al. WHO's new end TB strategy. Lancet. 2015;**385**(9979):1799-1801

[76] Albert H, Nathavitharana RR, Isaacs C, Pai M, Denkinger CM, Boehme CC. Development, roll-out and impact of XPERT MTB/RIF for

tuberculosis: What lessons have we learnt and how can we do better? EurRespir Journal. 2016;**48**(2):516e25

[77] World Health Organisation. Global Tuberculosis. Geneva: World Health Organisation; 2015b

[78] Barrera E, Livchits V, Nardell E. F-a-s-t: A refocused, intensified, administrative tuberculosis transmission control strategy. The International Journal of Tuberculosis and Lung Disease. 2015;**19**:381e4

[79] Fox GJ, Schaaf HS, Manalakas A, Chiappini E, Zumla A, Marais BJ. Preventing the spread of multidrug-resistant tuberculosis and protecting contacts of infectious cases. Clinical Microbiology and Infection. 2017;**23**(3):147-153

[80] Lönnroth K, Migliori GB, Abubakar I, D'Ambrosio L, de Vries G, Diel R, et al. Toward tuberculosis elimination: An action framework for low-incidence countries. The European Respiratory Journal. 2015;**45**:928-952

[81] Sotgiu G, D'Ambrosio L, Centis R, Bothamley G, Cirillo DM, De Lorenzo S, et al. TB and M/XDR-TB infection control in European TB reference centres: The Achilles' heel? The European Respiratory Journal. 2011;**38**:1221-1223

[82] Sotgiu G, Mauch V, Migliori GB, Benedetti A. Evidence-based agreed-upon health priorities to remedy the tuberculosis patient's economic disaster. The European Respiratory Journal. 2014;**43**:1563-1566

[83] D'Ambrosio L, Dara M, Tadolini M, Centis R, Sotgiu G, van der Werf MJ, et al. Tuberculosis elimination: Theory and practice in Europe. The European Respiratory Journal. 2014;**43**:1410-1420

[84] Falzon D, Jaramillo E, Schünemann HJ, Arentz M, Bauer M, Bayona J, et al. WHO guidelines for the programmatic management of drug-resistant tuberculosis: 2011 update. The European Respiratory Journal. 2011;**38**:516-528

[85] Schito M, Migliori GB, Fletcher HA, McNerney R, Centis R, D'Ambrosio L, et al. Perspectives on advances in tuberculosis diagnostics, drugs, and vaccines. Clinical Infectious Diseases. 2015;**61**(Suppl. 3):S102-S118

[86] Bayer R, Wilkinson D. Directly observed therapy for tuberculosis: History of an idea. Lancet. 1995;**345**:1545e8

[87] RNTCP. Guidelines for use of bedaquiline in RNTCP PMDT India. 2017. Available from: http://www.tbcindia.nic.in [Accessed: August 30, 2017]

[88] Kamat SR, Dawson JJ, Devadatta S, et al. A controlled study of the influence of segregation of tuberculous patients for one year on the attack rate of tuberculosis in a 5-year period in close family contacts in South India. Bulletin of the World Health Organization. 1966;**34**:517e32

[89] Lienhardt C, Cook SV, Burgos M, et al. Efficacy and safety of a 4-drug fixed-dose combination regimen compared with separate drugs for treatment of pulmonary tuberculosis: The Study C randomised controlled trial. JAMA. 2011;**305**:1415-1423